A Textbook for Dental Surgery Assistants

A Textbook for
Dental Surgery Assistants

3rd edition

S. F. Parkin MDS (Lond), FDSRCS (Eng)
Senior Lecturer in Children's Dentistry,
    Clinical Tutor, University College and
    Middlesex School of Dentistry, London
Honorary Consultant, University College
    Hospital Dental Hospital, London

Janet R. Oakeley
Registered Dental Surgery Assistant
City and Guilds' Technical Teacher's
    Certificate (now FAETC)
Formerly Tutor to the Dental Surgery Assistants
    at University College Hospital Dental
    Hospital, London

Wolfe Publishing Ltd

Published by
Wolfe Publishing Ltd
Brook House
2–16 Torrington Place
London WC1E 7LT

Reprinted 1993, by Clays Ltd, St Ives plc

First published in 1973 by Faber and Faber Limited. Revised
reprint 1977. Second edition 1983, revised reprint 1986. Third
edition 1989.

ISBN 0 7234 1838 1

For full details of all Wolfe titles please write to Wolfe Publishing
Ltd, Brook House, 2–16 Torrington Place, London WC1E 7LT,
England.

A CIP Catalogue record for this book is available from the British Library.

Contents

Preface to the Third Edition

This book is intended for dental surgery assistants at all stages of their career, but it should be of particular interest to those in training. We have aimed to provide a basic account of the theory and practice of the various branches of dentistry for use during the initial period of learning basic skills and gaining experience at the chairside, and also as an aid to revision. In selecting the material included we have paid close attention to the course of study suggested by the British Examining Board for Dental Surgery Assistants in preparation for the National Certificate.

This third edition has been extensively revised to include much new material and illustrations. Changes in terminology, materials, drugs and techniques are constantly occurring in modern dentistry as research continues to increase the scope of our knowledge and practice. Where possible we have tried to indicate the specific areas in which these changes are taking place: as we say, 'the trained dental surgery assistant owes it to herself and her profession to keep alert and up to date.'

We wish to acknowledge our profound debt to all those from whom we have learnt and to those whose work and research over the years have advanced modern dentistry to its present stage.

We are most grateful to the many friends and colleagues who have read sections of our manuscript and have helped us by giving valuable constructive criticism. So many people have assisted us in this way that we cannot begin to name them all here.

We thank our artists, Mrs Audry Besterman, Ashley S. Lupin and John M. Perkins for providing us with such excellent illustrations and for their meticulous attention to detail. We also thank Miss J. R. Blowers, Tutor to Dental Surgery Assistants, for her help and advice. We are indebted to Miss J. Vaughan, Senior DSA, and Mr Charles Day, chief photographer, University College and Middlesex Dental School, for new photographs of instruments and of DSAs carrying out procedures.

We are also indebted to the Amalgamated Dental Co Ltd for their permission to reproduce numerous illustrations of instruments from their catalogues and to Messrs KaVo DMI for generously allowing us to use illustrations of handpieces from their comprehensive range.

We are particularly grateful to the Examining Board for Dental Surgery

Assistants for permission to reproduce a selection of examination questions from recent papers.

We are most grateful to Mr Roger Osborne, Medical and Nursing Editor, Faber and Faber, whose encouragement and painstaking care have contributed so much to this edition.

Finally, we again give our special thanks to our families without whose patience, tolerance and support we would not have found the time or endurance to write this book at all.

S.F.P. and J.R.O.
1989

The Dental Profession

INTRODUCTION

Dentistry, in one form or another, has been practised throughout history, for toothache has always been one of the worst discomforts of mankind. Treatment was crude and of limited extent until medical science began to supplant ignorance.

For many centuries dentistry in Europe was mainly confined to the extraction of teeth until, in the 18th century, men like the French dentist Pierre Fauchard (1678–1761), author of the authoritative book *The Surgeon Dentist*, and John Hunter (1728–1793), in London, began to lay the foundations of modern dentistry.

Thus the dental surgeon replaced the ancient tooth drawer and dental science and practice developed rapidly. Dentistry became a discipline requiring its own course of study when the Medical Act of 1858 was passed, and the Royal College of Surgeons of England instituted an examination and diploma in dental surgery. Soon the established universities began to offer degrees in dental surgery.

The Dentists' Act 1921

With more people becoming dentists Parliament passed the Dentist's Act of 1921 which made it illegal for unregistered persons to practice dentistry. The General Dental Council only accepted names for the Dentists' Register of those practitioners who fulfilled certain stringent qualifications regarding training. Thus the practice of dentistry was controlled, and high standards of professional education and conduct among dentists were promoted.

The evolution of the dental surgery assistant (DSA)

Chairside assistants were of various standards throughout Britain until the Association of British Dental Surgery Assistants was founded in 1940 with the objects of protecting and furthering the interests of those assisting dental surgeons. An examination was introduced in 1947 and there are now training programmes available at all major dental hospitals and some colleges of further education. The status of the DSA is continually being raised and there is a growing awareness in the dental profession that the use of the trained chairside assistant is an essential part of dental practice. She is no longer a 'housekeeper' but a member of the dental team, serving dentistry in many ways – on the telephone, at the chairside, in the laboratory, in the office, meeting new patients, educating the patient, dealing with radiographs and, on her dental surgeon's behalf, the DSA is a goodwill ambassadress at all times. The procedures that a DSA may perform are determined by the British Dental Association's guidelines; in practice the duties of the DSA will depend on her particular qualifications, experience and the specific needs of her employer. The Association of British Dental Surgery Assistants aims to improve the training and career opportunities of its members and to gain the best advantage and benefits from qualifications. In 1964 a voluntary National Register of Dental Surgery Assistants was established, compiled by a joint committee of representatives from the British Dental Association and the Association of British Dental Surgery Assistants, listing all those who have passed an approved examination.

THE MODERN DENTAL PROFESSION

The governing bodies of the dental profession are the General Dental Council, the examining bodies (Universities and Royal Colleges) and the Department of Health which is responsible for the National Health Service.

The General Dental Council (GDC) ensures the standards of dental training and practice. Only those whose names appear on the dental register are permitted to practice. Once registered, any misdemeanour, for example, unprofessional conduct such as: (a) covering (associating with an unqualified person who is practising dentistry); (b) abusing the drug regulations; (c) abusing professional relationships; (d) falsifying certification of documents; and (e) advertising or canvassing for patients, may be disciplined by striking the practitioner's name from the Register. As far as the GDC regulations are concerned, a DSA counts as a non-registered person who is therefore forbidden to carry out dental treatment for patients apart from her normal duties of assisting a registered dentist at the chairside.

The educational and examining bodies such as the Royal Colleges and the Universities, monitored by the GDC to maintain standards, provide a series of examinations for registrable degrees for which undergraduate students study for up to five years at recognized schools.

The National Health Service (NHS) Act of 1946 which became operational on 5th July 1948, introduced a free health service into the United Kingdom for the first time. Today, the NHS is involved with most of the dental practice in Great Britain. It controls, monitors and finances dental practice carried out in general practice, hospital and community services. It demands certain specific obligations from the practitioner who is willing to undertake this work and sets the fees for items of service which may be paid directly from the NHS and partially from contributions by the individual patient at the time of treatment. (The dental surgeon is forbidden to carry out treatment both under the NHS and privately for a particular patient during one course of treatment.) It also requires prior permission before certain extensive courses of treatment are provided.

The NHS is managed from the Department of Health on behalf of the Minister of Health and the lines of communication, which vary from time to time because of reorganization, pass through the district health authority (DHA) to the district dental officer (DDO) who is in charge of the local community services, the family practitioner committee (FPC) in charge of general dental practice, and the dental estimates board (DEB) which deals with the monthly payments for completed courses of treatment and is also concerned with granting prior approval for certain types of treatment.

From time to time a sample of cases of completed treatment are called in for examination by another dental surgeon, employed by the DHSS, whose job is to ensure that the standards of treatment under the NHS are being maintained at all times. The DHSS dental officer may also examine patients if there is a problem about agreeing payment for unusual items of treatment. Up-to-date booklets providing detailed guidance with regard to NHS dental treatment, forms and documents are sent to all NHS practitioners from time to time and the DSA student should read one.

The *British Dental Association* (BDA) is a professional body which most qualified dental surgeons voluntarily join and which is alert to protect the interests of dental surgeons. Thus it is involved in negotiations on the profession's behalf with the government and other bodies and provides a network of professional groups throughout the United Kingdom which meet regularly for lectures, discussions and conferences. It publishes the *British Dental Journal* and maintains a professional library, reading room and museum at its headquarters in London where trained staff are available to advise members on all aspects of dentistry.

Dental practice can be carried out in a variety of circumstances, for example the commonest place is in general dental practice where the dental surgeon may be treating his patients under the rules of the NHS or by private arrangement with the individual patient. There are also occasions when domiciliary visits are necessary and the surgeon and assistant attend the patient in his own home.

The hospital services are provided by the NHS and here the dental surgeons hold a similar status to that of their medical and surgical colleagues, i.e. consultants with their registrars and house surgeons. Patients may be referred to such specialized hospital dental units when they present special problems of diagnosis and treatment – for example, major oral surgery, road traffic accidents, advanced orthodontic treatment and other specialties. At university dental schools which train both undergraduate and postgraduate students, the academic staff follow training similar to that of members of the hospital dental service, and clinical teaching staff usually hold honorary contracts in the NHS, which give the staffs parallel status. However, considerable importance is also attached to their teaching and research abilities, and published work.

The community services are also part of the NHS. Here the dental surgeon is a member of the salaried staff controlled by the district dental officer, whose surgery, staff and materials are provided for him. He is primarily responsible for treating children in local schools, but in addition cares for preschool children, expectant and nursing mothers, the homebound elderly, and the handicapped patients in his community. He is also concerned with preventive care and dental health education for the community. Operative work is generally carried out in permanent clinics, but in some areas the dentist may work in a specially equipped mobile clinic.

Some practices may be associated with industry, for example, within the environs of a large factory complex or a large multiple department store, so that the employees lose the minimum of time having treatment, and their dental welfare is ensured.

Within the armed forces dental surgeons join as commissioned officers and provide dental care for servicemen and their families.

Dental team

The dental team, working together to provide dental care for their patients as efficiently as possible, is always headed by the dental surgeon with his DSA, and in addition may also include the receptionist, other DSAs, the dental hygienist, the dental technician, and, in the community services, the dental health educator and the dental therapist.

Dental surgery assistants are employed in all areas of dentistry and have duties which are both varied and interesting, but their chief task is to assist the dentist and the patient before, during and after treatment. In the community dental service and in smaller general practices the duties of a DSA may well include the work of a receptionist (admitting patients, filing, making appointments, and handling general correspondence). In larger general practices where a receptionist is employed, the work of the DSA will be more concerned with helping the dental surgeon at the chairside in the provision of treatment.

Dental receptionists, although not directly concerned with the provision of dental treatment, contribute greatly to the smooth running of the practice which is of direct benefit to the patient. The dental receptionist is the first person patients see when they come to the surgery, or hear when they telephone, so tact, sympathy, a pleasant manner with an ability to put patients at their ease are all requirements of her work. She is also responsible for filing patients' notes, case histories and other paperwork necessary in dentistry – arranging appointments, sending out reminders, communicating with the NHS authorities and so on. Although there is no formal training, clerical and secretarial skills are obviously desirable.

Dental technicians are highly skilled craftsmen following four or five years' training, who construct dentures, crowns, bridges and orthodontic appliances, etc., according to the dental surgeon's requirements. They are important members of the dental team but do not provide treatment direct to members of the public. Many work in the general practice field but there are possibilities for specialization (for example, maxillofacial work, where the technician works in conjunction with a consultant oral surgeon to help restore the patient's face and oral structures after radical surgery, or following accident or deformity).

Dental hygienists, although not employed in all practices, have an important part to play in the dental team taking some of the dentist's workload. A hygienist who has completed a training course and passed the examination for the Certificate of Proficiency in Dental Hygiene is then entitled to entry in the Roll of Dental Hygienists and only those thus enrolled are permitted to practise under the direction of a dental surgeon. Duties include the scaling, cleaning and polishing of teeth, the application of preventive materials, such as fluoride and fissure sealants, to the teeth and instructing patients in the care of their mouths to keep teeth and gums healthy. With the demand for places to train as a hygienist so great, most schools expect applicants to have trained first as a DSA who may also have taken the Royal Society of Health's Diploma in Dental Health Education.

Dental health educationalists will have taken the Royal Society of Health's Diploma in Dental Health Education, and are employed in some cases to instruct patients and other members of the general public.

Dental therapists, after completing a 2-year course, are allowed to work only in the community service or hospital and may carry out dental treatment for children under the direction of a dental surgeon who will examine the children first and prescribe written treatment plans within certain defined limits. The dental therapist may scale and polish teeth, apply fluoride and fissure sealants, provide simple fillings and extract deciduous teeth under local infiltration anaesthesia, and conduct dental health education. She may often be helped in the surgery by a DSA.

Doctors may visit the practice as anaesthetists, and become members of the team to administer the necessary general anaesthetics for patients.

Other important visitors to the practice will include the representatives from dental companies and the engineers called in to repair and service existing dental equipment.

Useful addresses

Association of British Dental Surgery Assistants
DSA House
29 London Street
Fleetwood
Lancs
FY7 6JY

British Dental Association
64 Wimpole Street
London
WiM 8AL

General Dental Council
37 Wimpole Street
London
WiM 8DQ

The Royal Society of Health
RSH House
38a St Georges Drive
London
SWiV 4BH

CHAPTER ONE

Anatomy and Physiology

DEFINITIONS

Anatomy. This is the study of the form and structure of the body and of the relationships of its constituent parts to one another.

Physiology. This is the study of the function of the normal body as a whole and of its component parts and organs.

The cell. This is the microscopic unit from which all living organisms are built. Cells are composed of material called *protoplasm* which contains a watery solution (water = 70 per cent of the total cell volume) of proteins and small amounts of fats, carbohydrates, vitamins and salts.

Basically, an animal cell is a highly organized structure made up of a *nucleus* surrounded by a quantity of *cytoplasm* which is contained within the boundaries of a flexible *cell membrane*. The cell membrane is a permeable wall which allows selected materials to move in and out of the cell. The cytoplasm is concerned with the metabolism of the cell. The nucleus controls all cell processes and plays a vital part in cell division for it contains *genes* within the *chromosomes* which carry hereditary information. Although microscopically no two types of cells are identical, there is a common pattern of organization and generalizations can be made.

Cells are active, living units and demonstrate the basic characteristics of all living things: they use oxygen, they take in food for energy, growth and repair, they excrete waste products, at some stage they grow, they can reproduce (by cell division), they respond to outside stimuli and they can be killed.

TISSUES

In the human body the cells have *differentiated* into various types, each specialized to serve a particular purpose. This specialization means that cells are no longer capable of a separate existence but depend in turn on other groups of cells to collect oxygen and food and bring nutrition to them.

Tissues are made up of large numbers of identical cells which have developed to carry out a special function. They fall into four main groups.

Epithelial tissues. These serve as protective layers and membranes covering the surfaces of the body inside and out. For example, they form the skin and line the respiratory, digestive and urinary tracts. A secretory type of epithelium is found in *secretory glands* such as the salivary glands, the sweat glands and the tear glands.

Muscular tissues. These have the power of contraction. Three types are found in the body: *voluntary or striped*, for example the muscles of the limbs and the muscles of mastication; *involuntary, smooth or unstriped*, for example the muscles of the gut; and *cardiac*, the special muscle of the heart walls.

Connective tissues. These bind, connect and support the body and form a framework for the organs. *Areolar* tissue is a loose packing material. *Adipose* tissue contains fat. *Fibrous* tissue forms tendons and ligaments. *Bone*, the hardest connective tissue, forms the skeleton. *Cartilage* or gristle is found in various forms and hardnesses, for example, on the surfaces of joints, in the flexible external ear, in the intervertebral discs of the spine.

Nervous tissues. Nerve cells and their long processes form the brain, spinal cord and the nerves passing to all parts of the body. *Motor* or *efferent nerves* conduct (transmit) impulses from the brain and spinal cord to motivate all action in the tissues, for example, a muscle contraction. *Sensory* or *afferent nerves* conduct impulses to the brain from peripheral receptors, for example, the touch or thermal receptors in the skin. Many main nerve trunks are *mixed* and contain both sorts of nerve fibres.

An organ. This is any differentiated part of the body devoted to a special function; for example, tongue, eye, tooth, heart, lung or kidney.

ANATOMICAL TERMS

In anatomy the human body is studied and described as if it were standing in an upright position with the head erect and the eyes looking forward. An imaginary *median plane* runs vertically through the centre of the head, neck and trunk dividing them into left and right halves. The relative distances of structures from the median plane are described by the terms *medial* (nearer to) and *lateral* (further from). *Anterior* lies to the front or *ventral* side of the body and *posterior* to the back or *dorsal* side, while *superior* and *inferior* are used to indicate high and low positions. *Internal* and *external* describe the relative distances of a structure from the centre of a body cavity. *Superficial* and *deep* indicate the relative depths of structures from the surface of the body.

Systematic anatomy

For study purposes it is convenient to consider the different combinations of tissues, organs and structures according to the functions they perform.

1. The locomotor system: the skeleton, joints and muscles.
2. The circulatory system: the heart, blood vessels and blood.
3. The resipiratory system: the air passages and lungs.
4. The digestive system: the gastrointestinal tract and its associated organs.
5. The nervous system: the brain and peripheral nerves including the special senses.
6. The urogenital system: the urinary and reproductive systems.
7. The endocrine glands: the ductless glands which secrete hormones (substances causing activity at a distant site, for example, corticosteroids from the adrenal gland).

(This chapter studies only those sections of the general systems that are of importance to the dental surgery assistant's studies.)

LOCOMOTOR SYSTEM

Skeleton

This is the bony framework of the body, supporting the soft tissues and protecting the vital organs within the skull, vertebral canal, rib cage and pelvis. Many bones can move as levers about the joints in response to the action of attached muscles. The skeleton forms about 15 per cent of the total body weight.

Bone is a living tissue able to respond slowly to external influences, such as prolonged stress, by the remodelling action of bone-forming cells, *osteoblasts*, and bone-dissolving cells, *osteoclasts*. It acts as a storehouse of available calcium for the body.

Each bone is served by nutrient blood vessels and is also covered by a highly vascular tissue called the *periosteum*. The outer layer of a bone is very hard and dense, the *compact bone* or *cortex*, while the deeper internal layers are composed of lighter, spongy bone, the *cancellous bone*. Many bones have a central cavity, the *medullary cavity*, for example, within the shaft of a long bone of a limb, containing the fatty *bone marrow* which is the site of formation of red and white blood cells. The medullary cavity also serves to make the bone lighter.

The axial skeleton. This is made up of the skull, hyoid bone, vertebral column, ribs and sternum.

The appendicular skeleton. This is formed of the bones of the upper and lower limbs and the limb girdles (pelvis, collar-bones and shoulder-blades).

SKULL

This is made up of the eight bones of the *cranium* (the 'brain box') and the 14 bones of the *facial skeleton.*

Cranial bones
See Figs. 1/1, 1/2 and 1/3.

One *frontal* bone which forms the forehead and the upper margins of the eye sockets (the orbital cavities).

Two *parietal* bones which together form the roof and side walls of the cranium.

One *occipital* bone which forms the back and part of the floor of the cranium (the base of the skull). This bone is perforated by a large opening, the *foramen magnum* (foramen: an opening or hole, especially in bone) through which the lower part of the hind brain passes to join the spinal cord. On the external surface, on either side of this opening are the body facets, the *occipital condyles*, which support the skull at the top of the spinal column.

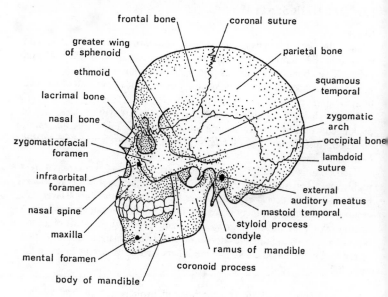

Fig. 1/1 Lateral aspect of the skull

Two *temporal* bones which form the lower side walls of the cranium. They contain the middle and inner parts of the hearing apparatus and also provide the fixed base for the *temporomandibular joint*.

One *sphenoid* bone which forms part of the floor of the cranium.

One *ethmoid* bone which lies at the front of the cranium forming the roof of the nasal cavity between the two orbits and is perforated by numerous holes (foramina) through which pass the *olfactory nerves* for the special sense of smell.

Facial skeleton

See Figs. 1/2 and 1/3, and Chapter 2.

Two *nasal* bones which form the bridge of the nose.

Two *zygomatic* bones, the cheek or malar bones which join the zygomatic processes of the temporal bones to form the *zygomatic arches*.

The *maxilla* which is formed of two halves and thus consists of two bones. It forms the lower border of the orbits, the sides of the nose aperture and also the upper jaw.

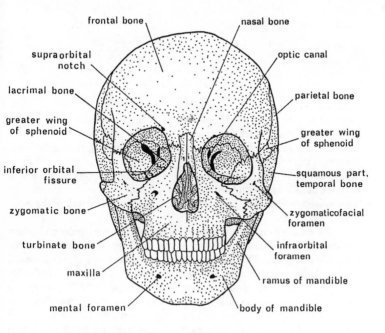

Fig. 1/2 Frontal aspect of the skull

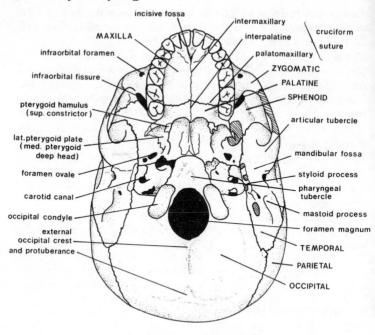

Fig. 1/3 Basal aspect of the skull

One *mandible* which forms the lower movable jaw and supports the teeth.

Two *palatine* bones which form part of the roof of the mouth.

Two *lacrimal* bones which contain the tear ducts and form part of the inner corners of the orbits.

One *vomer* bone which forms part of the nasal septum (the dividing wall between the left and right halves of the nasal cavity).

Two *inferior turbinate* bones which form part of the lateral wall of the nasal cavity.

With the exception of the mandible and some tiny bones in the middle ear (the auditory ossicles) all the bones of the skull are united by immovable joints called *sutures*. The maxillary, frontal, ethmoid and sphenoid bones contain hollow spaces, the *paranasal air sinuses*, which are lined with epithelium and are in communication with the nasal cavity. They serve to reduce the weight of the bony skull and also act as voice resonators. The bones of the skull are perforated by numerous foramina for the passage of nerves, blood vessels and other structures. The bones are rough and ridged and sometimes drawn into spines and processes where groups of muscles are attached to them, for example, the muscles of mastication and the muscles of facial expression.

Spine

This is also called the backbone or vertebral column and is a flexible column made up of 33 bones called *vertebrae*. There are seven *cervical* in the neck; the second cervical (axis) has the odontoid peg around which the atlas, or first cervical vertebra, moves when the head is rotated or in nodding. There are 12 *thoracic* associated with the ribs, five *lumbar* in the loins and, fused into two immovable groups, five *sacral* and four *coccygeal* vertebrae (the sacrum and the coccyx) which form the back of the pelvic girdle. The movable vertebrae are separated by intervertebral discs of fibrocartilage. Down the *vertebral canal* formed by the column of vertebrae and their processes runs the spinal cord from the brain giving off 31 pairs of spinal nerves which pass out through the intervertebral spaces.

Ribs

There are 12 pairs of ribs: seven 'true' ribs extending from the vertebral column to the *sternum* (breast bone), three 'false' ribs attached with cartilage to the sternum and two 'floating' ribs which are unattached in front. Together they form the *rib cage*.

Joints

These occur at the union of any two or more bones of the skeleton. They may be freely movable, for example the limbs, slightly movable, for example the vertebrae, or fixed, for example the skull or sacrum.

In movable joints the articulating bone surfaces are covered in smooth cartilage and the joint is contained within a fibrous capsule (the joint cavity) and held together by firm ligaments. The inside of the joint cavity is lined with a *synovial membrane* which secretes a lubricating fluid. Movable joints are subclassified by the mode of action, for example hinge, ball and socket, sliding and pivot joints.

Skeletal muscles

These are the contractile groups of striped muscle which cause bodily movement under the voluntary control of the nervous system. They are usually attached at each end: the *origin* is the end which remains stationary when the muscle contracts while the *insertion* attachment is drawn towards it. Muscle attachments may be to bone, cartilage, ligaments or skin. Strong movements require large muscles or groups of muscles working together. Muscles tend to work in opposition to other groups of muscles and by a fine balance of contraction and relaxation between them, delicate, controlled movements can be made. Muscles are generally described according to their shape, position, direction of movement or function.

CIRCULATORY SYSTEM

This system comprises the heart, blood vessels and the lymphatics.

Heart
See Fig. 1/4.
This is a hollow muscular pump which provides the motive power for the passage of blood to the tissues. It lies in the centre and slightly to the left of the mid-line of the chest. It is divided into left and right sides by the *septum*, each side being further divided into two chambers, the upper *atrium* and the lower, thicker-walled *ventricle*. The atria communicate with the ventricles through openings guarded by valves; on the right side the three-valved *tricuspid valve* and on the left the two-valved *mitral valve*. The right ventricle pumps blood to the lungs through the semilunar *pulmonary valve* while the left ventricle pumps blood to the rest of the body via the *aortic valve*. (On average the heart pumps 70ml of blood 70 times a minute for 70 years.)

Arteries carry blood away from the heart to the tissues. *Veins* carry blood

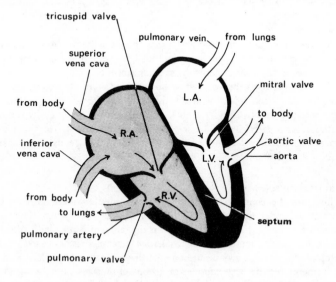

Fig. 1/4 The heart. The right atrium and the right ventricle are shaded to indicate that the blood they contain has not been oxygenated

toward the heart from the tissues (see also pages 18 and 126). *Capillaries* are very fine blood vessels in the tissues which link the arteries and the veins and through their walls allow nourishment, oxygen, waste products, and so on to be interchanged between the blood and the tissue fluid. *Lymphatics* are small vessels which act as a drainage system to carry away some of the fluid (lymph) which has exuded from the capillaries and, filtering it through the lymphatic glands, return it to the blood vessels in the thorax. They play an important part during inflammation.

CIRCULATION OF THE BLOOD
See Fig. 1/5.

Systemic circulation
Blood is pumped from the left ventricle of the heart into the *aorta*. In turn the aorta splits into smaller arteries and these subdivide further to serve all parts of the body. (The first branches from the aorta, the *coronary* arteries, serve the heart muscle itself.) The walls of the arteries are muscular and this helps to maintain the *blood pressure*. The pumping action of the heart causes pulsations in the arterial blood and this pulse can be felt in superficial

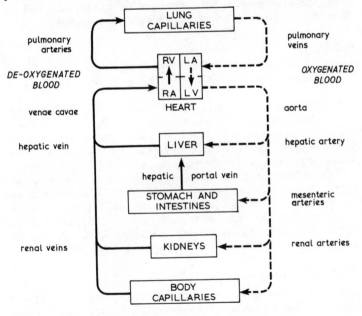

Fig. 1/5 The circulation of the blood (diagrammatic)

arteries such as those in the wrist. After passage through terminal *arterioles* into the capillaries, the blood flows back to the heart through the veins which empty through the *venae cavae* into the right atrium.

Pulmonary circulation

The returned systemic blood is pumped from the right atrium through to the right ventricle and thence out through the pulmonary artery to the lungs and into the pulmonary capillaries for gaseous exchange of oxygen and carbon dioxide. The oxygenated blood is returned to the left atrium via the pulmonary veins and is pumped through the left ventricle again.

Portal circulation

Blood from the stomach and gut, containing nutrient materials, is collected in the portal vein and transported directly to the liver. In addition the liver also has its own hepatic artery from the systemic circulation.

Renal circulation

Blood passes via the renal arteries to the kidneys where complex filtration occurs, the waste products being eliminated through the urine and the filtered blood returned to the general circulation via the renal veins.

Blood

This is a 'fluid tissue' made up of liquid blood plasma and its contained cells, a total of about 5 litres in an adult. Blood cells are of different types:

Red cells (erythrocytes). There are 3.9 to 6.5 $\times$ 10^{12}/litre of blood. These cells are very elastic and can accommodate themselves to the shape and dimensions of the narrowest vessels of the blood vascular system. They contain a protein complex, *haemoglobin*, concerned with the transport of oxygen. *Anaemia* means lack of haemoglobin.

Plasma contains substances which cause foreign red cells to stick together (agglutinate) and great care has to be taken if blood is transferred from one patient to another (transfusion) to make sure that they both belong to compatible *blood groups*. (Broadly, the groups are A, B, AB and O. A plasma agglutinates B cells, B plasma agglutinates A. AB plasma, 'the universal recipient', has no agglutinins and O, 'the universal donor', has both.)

White cells (leucocytes). These amount to 5.0 to 10.0 $\times$ 10^9/litre.

Granulocytes and polymorphonuclear leucocytes form 70 per cent of the total leucocytes. They are subdivided into neutrophils, eosinophils and basophils according to their staining reactions. The 'polymorphs' are mobile cells which deal with infection and invading bacteria and remove injured or dead tissue cells, usually by engulfing and digesting the undesirable material.

Lymphocytes form 25 per cent of the total white cells and take part in the defence mechanism and increase in numbers in chronic infection.

Monocytes form 5 per cent of the total white cells and may also play a part in the defence against chronic infection.

Platelets (thrombocytes). There are 2.5 to 3.5 × 10^{11}/litre. They have an important role in blood coagulation – the haemostatic mechanism.

Plasma. This is concerned with the transport of the blood cells and itself contains many dissolved materials including fibrinogen, the protein concerned with coagulation, and *antibodies* which provide immunity to specific organisms or toxins.

Coagulation. When blood is shed from a vessel, it sets into a jelly (blood clot) within 5 minutes (the clotting time). This jelly is formed by a complex chemical action between factors in the platelets and in the plasma whereby countless microscopic threads of *fibrin* are formed which entangle the cells. The jelly contracts and the defibrinated *serum* (a clear yellowish fluid) is exuded. This coagulation mechanism renders the circulation system 'self-sealing' following injury to a blood vessel and is the first stage in repair.

Functions of blood

1. The transport of oxygen to the tissues.
2. The transport of nutrients to the tissues.
3. The transport of waste materials and carbon dioxide from the tissues.
4. Assistance in the defence mechanism against infection and injury.
5. The transport of chemicals and hormones to the tissues.
6. Assistance in the distribution of heat throughout the body, and temperature control.
7. Coagulation and sealing of injuries to the circulatory system.

RESPIRATORY SYSTEM
See Fig. 1/6.

Oxygen is required for most of the chemical reactions in the body and in the production of heat and energy, carbon dioxide being produced as a waste product. *Respiration* means taking in oxygen and passing out carbon dioxide. The respiratory system is composed of the lungs, air passages and the mechanisms for expanding and contracting the walls of the thoracic cavity to *inspire* (draw in) and *expire* (breathe out) the air. During inspiration, air (which contains about 21 per cent oxygen) is drawn in through the *nose* where

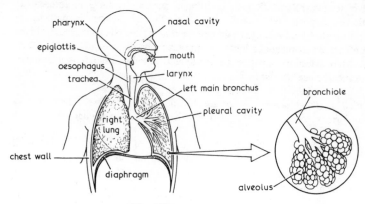

Fig. 1/6 Respiratory system

it is warmed and moistened before passing on through the *nasopharynx* and the *larynx*, between the vocal cords, down the *trachea* (windpipe, held open by rings of cartilage), through the smaller branching *bronchi* and via the small terminal *bronchioles* into the *alveoli* (air sacs) of the lungs. Once here the air is brought into close contact with a rich network of blood capillaries. The haemoglobin of the red cells, having a great affinity for oxygen, is converted to *oxyhaemoglobin* and carried back through the pulmonary veins to be passed on to the rest of the body, via the systemic circulation, where the oxygen is given up in the tissues. At the same time, deoxygenated haemoglobin and carbon dioxide are brought back to the lungs so that the carbon dioxide can be passed out from the capillaries through the air sac walls. (Note that except in the pulmonary circulation, arteries carry bright red 'oxygenated' blood to the tissues and veins carry dark red 'deoxygenated' blood from them.)

The expired air contains about 16 per cent oxygen (thus having lost about 5 per cent to the body) and now contains an increase of about 4 per cent of carbon dioxide.

The thoracic cavity which contains the lungs surrounded by a serous membrane, the *pleura*, is expanded by the action of muscles which raise the ribs and also by the depression of the *diaphragm*, a muscular sheet that separates the thorax from the abdomen. Expiration is usually achieved passively by an elastic 'recoil'. The respiratory cycle is mainly under the control of the respiratory centres of the brain which monitor the carbon dioxide levels in the circulating blood, but it is also under voluntary control for periods, such as breath-holding and during speech.

DIGESTIVE SYSTEM

See Fig. 1.7.

This system is concerned with the taking in (ingestion) of food and its preparation and breakdown for assimilation by the body. The *alimentary canal* is comprised of the mouth, pharynx and oesophagus above the diaphragm and the stomach, the small intestine (duodenum, jejunum and ileum) and large intestine (colon) and rectum below it.

Food

The body requires food for growth and repair and also to provide fuel for heat and energy. Foods contain a variety of important components.

1. Proteins. These are found in meat, eggs, cheese, and beans, and can be broken down to their basic *amino acids* which are important body-tissue building and repair materials.

2. Carbohydrates (*sugars, starches*). These provide the body with heat and energy. Once assimilated they may be stored in the liver and muscles in the form of *glycogen*.

3. Fats. These are contained in milk, butter, animal fat, olive oil, and other fats, and, like carbohydrates, are fuel foods. Fat may be stored in the body in the adipose tissue.

4. Mineral salts. The body tissues require adequate amounts of certain basic elements, in the form of soluble salts, including sodium, potassium, calcium, magnesium, phosphorus, sulphur, iron and iodine plus minute amounts of manganese, copper, zinc, and other trace elements.

5. Vitamins. These are essential food factors required for life, health and growth. Vitamins A, D, E and K are *fat-soluble* while B_1, B-complex and C are *water soluble*.

Vitamin A is found in fish liver oils, dairy products and carrots. A deficiency of this vitamin in the diet leads to night-blindness and a 'dry-eye' condition (xerophthalmia).

Vitamin D is found in fish liver oils and milk and is produced by the exposure of the skin to sun or ultraviolet rays. It is essential for the formation of sound bones and teeth. Deficiency causes soft-bone deformities (rickets) in infants and children.

Vitamin E, found in green vegetables, lettuce and wheatgerm, is essential for normal reproduction.

Vitamin K is found in spinach, cabbage, green foods and some cereals, and

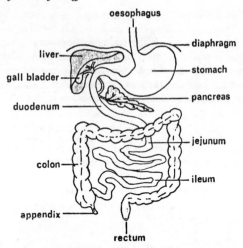

Fig. 1/7 Digestive system (below the diaphragm)

is necessary for the formation of a blood-coagulation factor (prothrombin). Deficiency leads to a bleeding (haemorrhagic) tendency.

Vitamin B_1, found in yeast and cereals, is essential for carbohydrate metabolism.

Vitamin B-complex is found in liver, yeast, wheatgerm and egg-yolk; a deficiency may lead to skin inflammation (dermatitis), cracks around the lips and nose, eye infections and anaemia.

Vitamin C is found in fruit, especially citrus fruits, tomatoes, blackcurrants and fresh vegetables; it is essential for the formation of connective tissues and their products, such as teeth and bones. Deficiency causes *scurvy* with bleeding from the mucous membranes and gingivae, beneath the skin and in the joint cavities with progressive anaemia, weakness and death if not treated over a period of many weeks.

6. Water. This is essential for the processes of digestion and excretion, to maintain the fluid balances of the tissues and to assist in temperature regulation (for example, sweating).

Digestion
Digestion is the process of mechanically and chemically breaking down food and simple compounds suitable for absorption into the body. The process may be divided into four stages:

1. Ingestion and mastication. Food is taken into the mouth and chewed (masticated) between the teeth, being held there by the action of the lips, tongue and cheeks. As the food is crushed and broken up it is mixed with saliva from the salivary glands which have been stimulated by the sight, smell and taste of the food. *Saliva*, a mixed secretion from the three pairs of salivary glands and the small mucous glands of the mucous membrane, contains the digestive enzyme, *ptyalin*, which converts starches to sugars. (An enzyme is an agent, usually a protein, that has the property of accelerating a chemical reaction.) The saliva is mixed with the food, thoroughly moistening it and lubricating it for swallowing. The mass of food is now moulded into a ball or *bolus*.

2. Deglutition (swallowing). This has three stages, the first voluntary, the other two involuntary.

(a) The bolus is placed at the back of the tongue, the teeth are brought together and the tongue raised upwards and backwards to project the food into the pharynx.
(b) The bolus is now passed rapidly through the upper part of the pharynx, which is the region common to both the respiratory and digestive passages. The tongue remains in position to prevent the food returning to the mouth. The soft palate is raised to touch the back of the pharynx and stop the food from entering the nose. The larynx is raised up until it lies under the protection of the epiglottis at the base of the tongue and respiration is inhibited for a moment so that the food cannot enter the trachea. The bolus is gripped by the constrictor muscles of the pharynx and passed into the oesophagus (gullet).
(c) The oesophagus is a muscular tube that conducts the food down to the stomach by a wave of muscular contraction (*peristalsis*) that is partly aided by gravity. The food is thus carried through the chest and down through the diaphragm into the abdomen, entering the stomach through a ring of muscle, the *cardiac sphincter*, that acts as a valve guarding the entrance.

3. Digestion and absorption. In the stomach the food is mixed with the gastric juices by the muscular contractions of the stomach walls. *Gastric juice* is secreted by special cells in the stomach lining. It is highly acid and contains special enzymes including *pepsin*, *rennin* and *lipase* which act upon the proteins and fats.

At intervals the acid contents of the stomach, the *chyme*, are released into the upper part of the small intestine, the *duodenum*. The duodenal contents soon become alkaline by the action of digestive fluids brought to the duodenum by ducts from the liver and pancreas. *Bile* from the liver is alkaline and also emulsifies fats. *Pancreatic juice* contains the enzymes *amylase*, *lipase* and *trypsin* which act on carbohydrates, fats and proteins respectively. *Succus entericus*, the intestinal juice secreted by tiny glands in the small intestine wall also contains *erepsin*, an enzyme which acts upon proteins, and *invertase*, *maltase* and *lactase* which deal with sugars. The fluid food is passed along the intestine by peristaltic waves of muscular contraction which are preceded by corresponding waves of relaxation. By now all the usable food material has been broken down to its final state ready for absorption. This takes place through the walls of the small intestine (duodenum, jejunum and ileum). The walls are raised into tiny finger-like processes, *villi*, which greatly increase the absorbing surface of the intestine. The villi are well served with blood capillaries and lymphatics, here called *lacteals*. The food products are taken either directly into the blood-stream and carried straight to the liver for storage or further chemical processes or, in the case of fat, into the lacteal and hence into the lymphatic system and on to the general circulation.

4. Excretion. The unusable residue and waste products pass on into the large intestine where water and salts are removed and the more solid *faeces* are passed into the *rectum* for elimination through the *anus*.

(The term *excretion* means the discharge of waste materials from the body. The kidneys filter the blood and eliminate water, salts and other end-products of metabolism via the urine. The lungs excrete carbon dioxide and water and can eliminate inhalation anaesthetic agents. The skin excretes water and salts in the perspiration. The saliva can also excrete certain materials, such as mercury and lead, in cases of poisoning.)

NERVOUS SYSTEM

This is the communication system of the body. The brain, spinal cord and nerves are composed of nerve cells and their processes. Each nerve cell or *neurone* has many processes, *dendrites*, for collecting impulses, and a single process, the *axon*, for passing the impulse on from the cell body. The nervous system is composed of millions of linked neurones.

The system, is divided into two subsystems: the *central nervous system* (the brain, spinal cord and peripheral nerves) and the *autonomic nervous system* (the sympathetic and parasympathetic systems).

Central nervous system
Brain. This is the control centre for the whole body. It weighs about 2 per cent of the total body-weight and requires a litre of oxygenated blood every minute. Lack of oxygen for more than 10 seconds results in loss of consciousness and if this deficiency continues for more than 4 minutes permanent brain damage will result. The brain is covered by the vascular *meninges* and these in turn are covered by a tough protective membrane, the *dura mater*.

L. SMITH

Peripheral nervous system. This system connects the brain to all parts of the body. It is composed of two kinds of nerves, the *efferent nerves* which carry messages from the brain and spinal cord to various parts of the body, for example, motor impulses to voluntary muscles; and *afferent nerves* which relay messages back to the brain for interpretation, for example, sensations of pain or temperature changes from the skin.

Cranial nerves. These originate from the brain within the cranium. Some are *sensory*, some are *motor* and some are *mixed* nerves.

	Name	*Type*	*Distribution and function*
1st	Olfactory	Sensory	Olfactory mucous membrane of the nose: SMELL
2nd	Optic	Sensory	Retina of eye: SIGHT
3rd	Oculomotor	Motor	Eyeball muscles
4th	Trochlear	Motor	Eyeball muscles
5th	Trigeminal	Mixed	Sensory to forehead, face, nose, mouth, teeth, etc.; three branches: (i) ophthalmic, (ii) maxillary, (iii) mandibular. Motor to muscles of mastication
6th	Abducens	Motor	Eyeball muscle
7th	Facial	Mixed	Sensory to anterior two-thirds of tongue: TASTE. Motor to muscles of facial expression
8th	Auditory	Sensory	From the cochlea: HEARING. From the semicircular canals via the vestibular nerve: BALANCE
9th	Glossopharyngeal	Mixed	Sensory from the tongue: TASTE. Motor to muscles of the pharynx
10th	Vagus	Mixed	Supplies the pharynx, larynx, trachea, bronchi, lungs, heart, stomach, oesophagus and upper part of the intestine
11th	Accessory	Motor	Muscles of pharynx, layrnx and muscles in the neck and shoulder
12th	Hypoglossal	Motor	Muscles of the tongue

The 5th and 7th nerves (the trigeminal and facial) are described in more detail in Chapter 2, pages 46–7.

Spinal cord. This lies within the vertebral canal and gives off 31 pairs of mixed spinal nerves which serve all parts of the body, either by direct communication with the brain or by reflex action. Reflex actions are involuntary movements, for example, when the hand is pricked with a pin it is withdrawn rapidly without conscious thought.

Autonomic nervous system

This system is connected with the brain and central nervous system but is devoted to involuntary action which takes place in, for example, the intestines, the blood vessels, heart and lungs. The sympathetic and parasympathetic systems which together make up the autonomic system, work in opposition to one another, the action of one stimulating an organ while the action of the other inhibits it, for example, the heart rate and force are increased by the sympathetic and decreased by the parasympathetic; the bronchi are relaxed by the sympathetic and contracted by the parasympathetic. In this way a precise adjustment or tone between activity and rest can be maintained.

Sympathetic system. This is a double chain of ganglia (groups of nerve cells) which lie in front of the vertebral column from the base of the skull to the pelvis and send branches to the heart, blood vessels, stomach, intestines, muscles and skin and most other organs.

Parasympathetic system. This operates through the 3rd, 7th, 9th and 10th cranial nerves to the eyes, salivary glands, and all over the body via the vagus nerve and through the sacral region of the spinal cord. Its distribution is similar to the sympathetic.

USEFUL AVERAGES

Temperature

Usually taken with a glass/mercury clinical thermometer, but occasionally with a reactive strip or electronic digital system. *Normal temperature* is 36.8–37.2 °C (98–99 °F). When taken in the mouth the patient must keep his/her lips closed and breathe through the nose. The temperature rises with fever, exercise, etc. and falls in shock.

Pulse rate

This reflects the heart rate and is taken by palpating (feeling) a superficial artery, for example, in the wrist (radial), or neck (carotid) for a full minute. *Normal pulse rate* is 60–80 beats per minute, normally faster in children. The pulse rate increases with excitement, anxiety, exercise, haemorrhage, etc. and in disease the strength and rhythm may alter.

Respiratory rate

This is taken by counting the number of respirations per minute. Each respiration consists of a complete in and out breathing cycle.
Normal respiratory rate is 16–18 times per minute, but it can be twice as fast in children.

The respiratory rate rises with increased bodily need for oxygen, for example, in anxiety, exercise, fever or severe chest or heart diseases.

Blood pressure

This reflects aspects of the cardiovascular system: pumping force of the heart, circulating blood volume, elasticity of blood vessels, etc. It is taken with a *sphygmomanometer* calibrated in millimetres of mercury (mmHg). An inflatable cuff or armband is wrapped around the reclining patient's upper arm and pumped up until the radial pulse cannot be felt. Then, listening through a *stethoscope* to the brachial artery in the arm below the cuff, the air is slowly released. Two sounds will be heard as the blood flows again, first a tapping sound, (the *systolic pressure*, when the heart contracts) then, as the air pressure falls, the sound suddenly becomes softer (the *diastolic pressure*, when the heart relaxes).

Average systolic pressure: 100–140 mmHg
Average diastolic pressure: 60–90 mmHg

The difference between the systolic and diastolic pressures is called the *pulse pressure*.

Systolic pressure averages vary with age, exercise, anxiety, and rest, and are higher in the elderly. They fall in shock and are raised in certain cardiovascular disorders such as essential hypertension.

CHAPTER TWO

Dental Anatomy and Physiology

Study note: The study of the shape of individual teeth and the bones of the upper and lower jaw is greatly simplified by referring to the actual structures. We would advise the student to collect and sterilize a set of extracted human teeth for study; to examine either a plastic or dried skull; to examine her own dental structures in a mirror, as well as those of patients undergoing treatment; and to feel the movement of her own jaws, i.e. the contraction of the facial and masticatory muscles and the temporomandibular joint.

TEETH

These are hard, mineralized structures which are set in bony sockets in the upper and lower jaws. Their main function is to masticate food and prepare it for swallowing. They also play an important part in the growth and final contour of the lower half of the face and are required for the clear articulation of certain sounds in speech.

A tooth consists of two main parts: the *crown* which is the part visible in the mouth and the *root* (or roots) which is the part set in the jaw. Where the crown and the root join, the tooth is usually constricted into the *neck* (the cervix or *cervical region*) (Fig. 2/1).

There are four main types of teeth: *incisors* or cutting teeth at the front of the mouth; *canines* ('eye teeth' or 'teeth such as dogs have'), at the corners of the mouth, which are used for gripping and tearing; *premolars* (bicuspids) which are not present in the child's primary dentition and *molars* or millstone teeth at the back of the mouth.

The teeth are set into the upper (maxillary) and lower (mandibular) alveolar processes (the special tooth-supporting bone) in curved arcades or *dental arches*.

Each tooth has four surrounding surfaces and a working edge or surface: *mesial*, nearest to the median plane; *distal*, furthest away from the median plane; *labial* or *buccal* nearest to the lips or cheek; *lingual* nearest to the tongue (in the upper jaw the term *palatal*, nearest to the palate, is generally used instead of *lingual*); *occlusal*, the working surface of molars and premolars; *incisal edge*, the cutting edge of incisors (Figs 2/2 and 2/3). The *proximal*

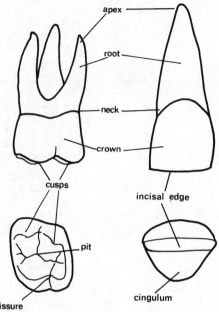

Fig. 2/1 External anatomy of teeth: (left) an upper molar; (right) an upper incisor

surfaces are those which lie against the adjacent teeth in the same arch, that is, the mesial and distal.

Cusps are the raised mounds on the occlusal surfaces of molars and premolars and raised lines are called *ridges*. *Fissures* are the line crevices between cusps. Small pinpoint depressions are called *pits*. The *contact area* of a tooth is where it touches the surface of an adjacent tooth in the same arch. A *cingulum* is the raised ridge prominent only on the palatal surface of upper incisors.

Each tooth is made up of four tissues – enamel, dentine, dental pulp and cementum (Fig. 2/4) – and is supported by the periodontal structures of the tooth socket.

Enamel

This is the hard, translucent, mineralized, insensitive material which covers the anatomical crown of the tooth. It is the hardest tissue in the body, composed mainly of calcium and phosphorus in the form of *hydroxyapatite* and containing only some 1 per cent of organic material. It is formed in microscopic *prisms* (or *rods*) joined by weaker *interprismatic substance* along

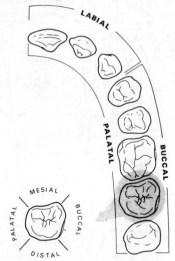

Fig. 2/2 Tooth surfaces in the maxilla

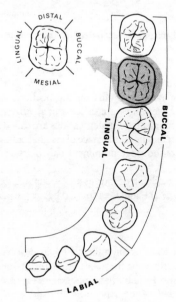

Fig. 2/3 Tooth surfaces in the mandible

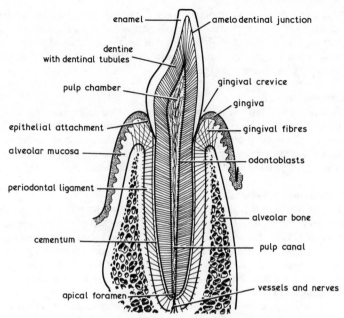

Fig. 2/4 A tooth and its component tissues

which the enamel may be sheared or fractured mechanically during cavity preparation. It is the thickest at the occlusal surface of the teeth.

Dentine
This is the yellowish, tough, slightly elastic material which forms the bulk of the tooth. In the crown it lies just beneath the enamel which it contacts at the *amelodentinal junction*. Dentine is mineralized but has about a 20 per cent organic content. It is traversed by fine *tubules* each containing a *fibril* or thread from the outer layer of pulpal cells, the *odontoblasts*. Thus dentine is sensitive, and with the pulp can react to moderate stimulation or injury but is vulnerable to strong chemicals or excessive heating during cavity preparation, etc. (Note: the *ivory* of an elephant's tusk is dentine.)

Dental pulp
This is the 'nerve' or soft tissue which occupies the pulp chamber of the crown and the root canal(s) within the dentine. The root canal communicates with the *periapical* (around the tip of the root) tissues through the *apical foramen* of the tooth. The pulp contains nerve fibres, blood vessels, lymphatics and connective tissue and is surrounded at its junction with the dentine

by the continuous layer of odontoblasts. The pulp gives the tooth vitality, nutrition and sensitivity; in the embryonic stages it is formative and forms the dentine; and it plays a defensive role in repairing damaged dentine by calcification and the formation of *secondary dentine* within the pulp chamber. The pulp gets smaller with age.

Cementum

This is the thin layer of material which covers the anatomical root of the tooth. It resembles bone in composition and serves to attach the periodontal fibres to the tooth. It protects the underlying dentine, reacts to compensate for occlusal stresses and strains by changing in thickness and may transmit a little nutrition to the tooth from the periodontal tissues.

Periodontal membrane

This is the ligament which attaches the tooth to the walls of the socket formed around it by the alveolar bone. It is composed of strong connective tissue fibres together with numerous cells and blood vessels, lymphatics and nerves. At the neck of the tooth these tissues merge with those of the gingivae and the periosteum of the bone. The principal fibres of the periodontal membrane are described according to their function and the direction in which they run.

The free gingival fibres from the cervical cementum together with *vertical fibres* from the alveolar crest or socket margin pass into the gum next to the tooth to keep it in firm contact with the tooth. *Transseptal fibres* run from one tooth to its neighbour, interdentally, and help to maintain the arch. The *circular ligament* and *horizontal fibres* pass from the alveolar crest region to the cervical cementum and stabilize the tooth against lateral stress. (These important fibres are the first to disintegrate in the onset of periodontal disease.) Below this level the major part of the ligament is composed of *oblique fibres* that pass obliquely upwards from the cementum in the direction of the alveolar crest. All these fibres serve to stabilize and cushion the tooth against masticatory strains. The nerve endings are sensitive to pressure and pain and thus give a general awareness of which teeth are in contact during mastication and protect the dental apparatus from excessive pressure, such as on a stone.

The width of the various regions of the periodontal membrane varies according to occlusal stress and it becomes thinner with age as the cementum thickens.

ALVEOLAR BONE PROCESSES

These processes of the maxilla and mandible form the tooth sockets which are closely adapted to the shape of the roots. The socket walls are perforated by numerous foramina which transmit blood vessels and nerves to the periodontal membrane and the tooth. The lining of the socket wall to which the periodontal fibres are attached is composed of slightly denser bone, the *lamina dura*, which can be identified on an intraoral radiograph. The alveolar bone adapts and remodels gradually in response to functional pressures.

THE GINGIVA

This is also called the 'gum' and is that part of the oral mucosa which surrounds the teeth. In health it is pale pink, slightly stippled on the surface and in close contact with the tooth. The *free gingiva* is separated from the tooth surface by the shallow *gingival crevice*. At the base of this crevice there is a firm *epithelial attachment* between the epithelial tissues and the tooth surface. (This attachment is destroyed in the first stages of pocket formation; see Chapter 11.) The interdental space is occupied by the *interdental papilla* of gingival tissue. The gingivae have a good blood supply and contain a high proportion of connective tissue.

ORAL MUCOSA

This lines the whole oral cavity and is composed basically of two layers: the *epithelium* and the underlying *connective tissues*. It contains numerous tiny mucous glands and is thickened in places of intensive masticatory wear, such as the palate (where it is raised in ridges, the *rugae*), and the gingivae. Over the surface of the tongue the mucosa is specialized to serve the sense of taste. The junction between the red margins of the lips and the external skin is called the *transitional zone*.

DEVELOPMENT OF THE TEETH AND JAWS

At an early stage in the development of the human embryo, the cells are differentiated into three layers: the *ectoderm*, which will form the external surface of the body and its derivatives including parts of the mouth, the salivary glands and enamel of the teeth and most of the central nervous system; the *endoderm* which gives rise to the alimentary canal and such things as the lungs and air passages; and the *mesoderm* which forms the remaining organs and tissues including the dentine, cementum and pulp of the teeth, the muscles and cardiovascular system.

The face and neck of the embryo begins to differentiate as early as five weeks *in utero* into the form of six primitive *visceral arches*, like those of a fish, in the wall of the foregut. The first of these arches, the *mandibular*, will go on to form the lower jaw, chin, the anterior two-thirds of the tongue and the muscles of mastication, carrying with it the mandibular division of the 5th trigeminal nerve. In addition, the maxilla, excluding the premaxilla, is developed from the maxillary processes of the mandibular arch. The second arch, the *hyoid*, forms the muscles of facial expression, etc., carrying with it the 7th facial nerve. The third arch forms the posterior part of the tongue and carries the 9th glossopharyngeal nerve fibres with it.

The tooth germ

This begins to form by a proliferation of ectodermal cells in the primitive mouth at about 6 weeks *in utero* (Fig. 2/5). The cells form a band, the *dental lamina*, around the jaw and at nine weeks little buds of cells appear, one for each primary tooth. These buds form into the bell-shaped *enamel organs* (which have an internal wall of enamel-forming cells, the *ameloblasts*) and stimulate the associated mesodermal cells to form *dental papillae* which will in turn form the dentine and dental pulp. Each tooth germ is contained inside a sac called the *dental follicle*. Offshoots from these tooth germs and a distal extension of the dental lamina make provision for the permanent tooth buds. Mineralization of the teeth begins at about 18 weeks, so that at birth a considerable part of the deciduous teeth is already calcified.

Eruption of teeth

This is not fully understood. It may be due to blood pressure, root growth, changes in the bone of the alveolar process or even the influence of the

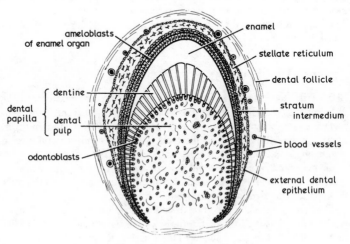

Fig. 2/5 A developing tooth

'ingrown' epithelial tissues trying to return to the surface. The tooth gradually rises to the surface and the epithelial remnants of the enamel organ (*Nasmyth's membrane*, the 'skin of the tooth') become attached to the surface epithelium at the gingival crevice as the tooth erupts into the mouth. This attachment recedes gradually until it rests on the amelocemental junction. Teeth commonly erupt before the apex of the root is fully formed and this is completed in conjunction with the formation of the final socket.

THE DENTITIONS

See Figs 2/6, 2/7 and 2/8.

There are two dentitions: the primary, deciduous or 'milk teeth' of the child (Fig. 2/6) and the permanent or secondary teeth (Fig. 2/7).

Primary dentition

See Fig. 2/6.

This consists of 20 teeth, five in each quadrant: two incisors, one canine and two molars. They are small teeth, set vertically in the alveolus, with whiter enamel than the permanent teeth. They have relatively barrel-shaped crowns with large pulps and slender tapering roots. The permanent premolar tooth germs lie between the divergent roots of the molars. The upper 1st molar has three cusps while the upper 2nd molar has four cusps. The lower 1st molar has four cusps and the lower 2nd molar has five cusps.

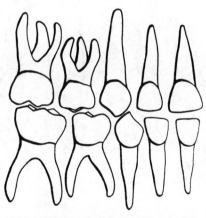

Fig. 2/6 The primary teeth (primary dentition)

Eruption and calcification table for primary teeth

	Calcification		Tooth erupts	Resorption begins	Tooth shed
	Begins (intrauterine)	Completed (after birth)			
1st incisor	18th week	18 months	6 months	3	7th year
2nd incisor			8 months	years	8th year
1st molar	20th week	20 months	12 months	before	9th year
canine	24th week	24 months	18 months	being	11th year
2nd molar			24 months	shed	10th year

Permanent dentition

See Fig. 2/7.

This consists of 32 teeth, eight in each quadrant: two incisors, one canine, two premolars and three molars.

Incisors. These are the chisel-shaped cutting teeth at the front of the mouth. They have one root and the crown is convex on the labial surface and concave on the palatal/lingual surface. The upper central incisor is larger than the others and may have a ridge on the palatal surface, near the cervical region, called the *cingulum*.

Canine tooth. This is also called the cuspid and is a strong, conical tooth more massive than an incisor, with a single root that is usually larger than any of the others in the mouth. The lower canine is smaller than the upper.

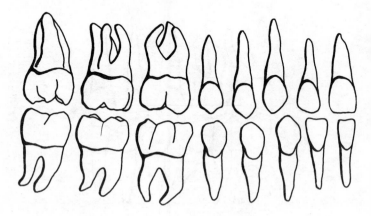

Fig. 2/7 The permanent teeth (permanent dentition)

Premolars. These are also called bicuspids and occupy a position between the canines and the molars. They have occlusal surfaces and cusps. The 1st upper premolar may have two roots but all the others have only one root. The lingual cusp on the lower 1st premolar is very small and care must be taken not to confuse this tooth with the canine.

Molars. These teeth have the largest occlusal surfaces; the upper molars have four cusps, the lower 1st molar has five cusps, the lower 2nd molar has four cusps and the lower 3rd molar has five cusps. The upper molar teeth each have three roots (mesiobuccal, distobuccal and palatal) while the lower molars each have two-roots (mesial and distal). The third molars, the 'wisdom teeth', may occasionally vary from this pattern of cusp and root numbers. Sometimes there is an additional palatal cusp on the upper first molars – the cusp of Carabelli.

Figure 2/8 illustrates how the primary and permanent dentitions overlap in the jaws.

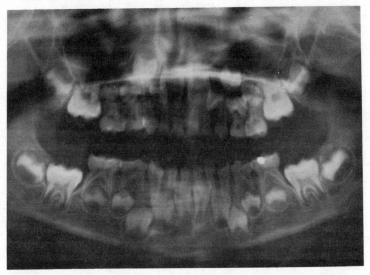

Fig. 2/8 Orthopantomogram showing how the mixed dentitions are related in the jaws

Eruption and calcification table for permanent teeth
(after Aitchison)

	Tooth erupts (years)	Calcification begins	Calcification completed
1. 1st incisor	7	for all teeth	
2. 2nd incisor	8	6 years before eruption	3 years after eruption
3. canine	11	except for canine	
4. 1st premolar	9	and 3rd molar	
5. 2nd premolar	10	when calcification	
6. 1st molar	6	begins 9 years	canine and 3rd
7. 2nd molar	12	before	molar completely
8. 3rd molar	18–24	eruption	calcified upon eruption

THE JAWS

Maxillae

See Figs 2/9, 2/10 and 2/11.

These together form the left and right halves of the upper jaw. Each bone supports the upper teeth, forms the hard palate (in conjunction with the palatine bone) and helps to make up the floor of the orbit and the floor and lateral wall of the nasal cavity. The maxilla has a pyramid-shaped body with four surfaces – anterior, posterior, nasal and orbital; and four processes – frontal, zygomatic, palatine and alveolar. The body of the maxilla encloses a large air cavity: the *maxillary air sinus* or *antrum*.

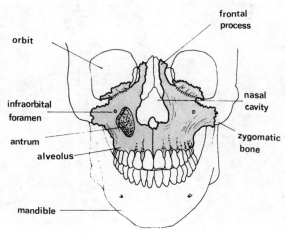

Fig. 2/9 Frontal aspect of the maxilla

Maxillary sinus. This communicates with the nasal cavity and is lined with ciliated, respiratory epithelium. The floor of the sinus lies in close relationship to the roots of the 1st and 2nd upper molar teeth and in some cases a large sinus may relate to all the molars and premolars. (This fact must be borne in mind during infections or extraction of these teeth.) The posterior wall is perforated by the dental canals carrying posterior superior dental vessels and nerves to the molar teeth.

Orbital surface. This forms part of the floor of the orbit and has a groove running forwards which carries the infraorbital nerve and artery down via the *infraorbital canal* to the *infraorbital foramen* to the surface of the face below the orbit (Fig. 2.10).

Anterior surface. This supports the cheek and carries three processes: the *frontal* which passes upwards on the medial aspect of the orbit and articulates with the frontal bone and the nasal bone; the *zygomatic* which articulates with the *zygomatic bone* (the cheek bone); and the *alveolar process* which supports the teeth.

Posterior surface. This bulges outwards and is directed backwards and laterally. It is perforated by the dental canals. At its lower part is the *maxillary tuberosity*, a rounded knob of bone that lies distally to the upper 3rd molar in the arch.

Nasal surface. This carries the opening of the antrum and forms part of the wall of the nasal cavity.

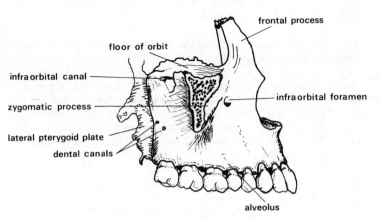

Fig. 2/10 Lateral aspect of the right maxilla

Palatal process. See Fig. 2/11. This articulates in the mid-line with the opposite maxilla and with the palatal bone posteriorly to form the hard palate. The palate is grooved at its posterior part to provide a channel for the *greater palatine vessels and nerve* as they run forward from the *greater palatine foramen.* Immediately behind the incisor teeth lies the *incisive fossa* which transmits the *long sphenopalatine nerve* and the *sphenopalatine artery.*

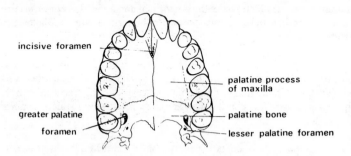

incisive foramen

palatine process of maxilla

greater palatine foramen

palatine bone

lesser palatine foramen

Fig. 2/11 Palatal aspect of the maxilla

Mandible. See Figs. 2/12 and 2/13. This is also called the lower jaw and is the largest and strongest bone of the face. It articulates on each side with the *glenoid fossa* of the temporal bone. It is formed of two parts: the horseshoe-shaped, curved, horizontal *body*; and the two broad, flattened *rami* which project upwards from the posterior ends of the body.

Body. This is composed of right and left halves which are fused in the mid-line at the *symphysis menti.*

External surface of the body. At the mid-line the chin is formed by the triangular *mental protuberance.* The depression above this protuberance is the *incisive fossa.* The *external oblique* line runs upwards and backwards from the margin of the mental protuberance to become the anterior border of the ascending ramus. Below and between the premolar teeth the *mental foramen* transmits the mental nerve and vessels.

Internal surface of the body. This is divided into two areas by the *mylohyoid ridge* which gives attachment to the mylohyoid muscle and runs obliquely down from behind the third molar to a point low down at the mid-line behind the symphysis menti. Just above this mid-line point are two pairs of small

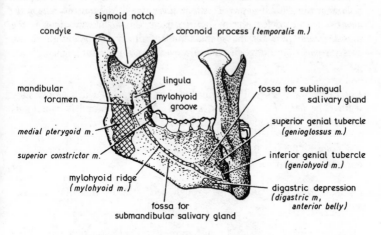

Fig. 2/12 The mandible from behind

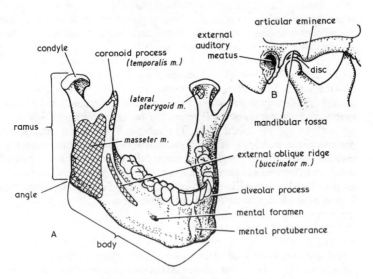

Fig. 2/13 The mandible from the front

tubercles, the *genial tubercles*, which are the origin of the *genioglossus* and *geniohyoid* muscles. Below the mylohyoid line near the symphysis lies the hollow of the *digastric depression* which gives rise to the *anterior belly of the digastric muscle*. Below the posterior part of the mylohyoid ridge is the *submandibular fossa* for the submandibular salivary gland and above the anterior part of the ridge lies the *sublingual fossa* for the sublingual salivary gland.

Upper border of the body. This forms the alveolar process which supports the teeth. The *lower border* is thick, smooth and rounded and is continuous behind with the thin lower border of the ramus.

The ramus. This is a flattened quadrilateral shape with two surfaces, four borders and two processes.

External surface of the ramus. This is roughened by the insertion of the *masseter muscle*.

Internal surface of the ramus. In the centre of this surface, at the level of the occlusal plane of the molar teeth, is the *mandibular foramen* through which pass the inferior dental nerve and vessels into the mandibular canal. Guarding the front of the foramen is a tongue of bone, the *lingula*, which gives attachment for the *sphenomandibular ligament*. A shallow *mylohyoid groove* (for the mylohyoid nerve and vessels) runs downwards and forwards for a short distance. Below this groove is an area roughened by the attachment of the *medial pterygoid muscle*.

Borders of the ramus. The *inferior border* is thin and rounded and in continuity with the body in front. Its junction with the *posterior border* forms the angle of the mandible. This posterior border is rounded and smooth and is surrounded by the *parotid gland*. The *anterior border* is continuous with the external oblique line of the body. The *superior border* has two important processes separated by a notch, the *sigmoid notch*. The anterior process is the thin triangular *coronoid process* which carries the insertion of the *temporalis muscle* on its internal and anterior surfaces. The posterior process carries the *condyle* which has a broad, strong, rounded head on a thin neck and forms the joint surface which articulates with the temporal bone.

Temporomandibular joint
See Fig. 2/13B.
This is a sliding-hinge joint which allows grinding movements of the jaws to take place. The *glenoid* or *mandibular fossa* of the temporal bone is an oblong concavity bounded anteriorly by a raised *articular eminence*. As the body of the

mandible moves downwards, the condyle slides forwards and downwards on to the eminence. The joint has a fibrocartilaginous *disc* which is more firmly attached to the condyle than the fossa. The joint is protected by the *capsular ligament* around the joint, strengthened by internal and external *lateral ligaments* and further reinforced by the *sphenomandibular ligament* (spine of the sphenoid to the lingula) and *stylomandibular ligaments* (styloid process to the posterior border of the ramus above the angle of the jaw).

MUSCLES OF MASTICATION
See Figs 2/14, 2/15 and 2/16.

Temporalis. This is a fan-shaped muscle. Its origin is the temporal fossa at the side of the cranium and its insertion the coronoid process of the mandible. It serves to elevate the mandible and also draw it backwards.

Masseter. This is a quadrilateral muscle in superficial and deep portions. It arises from the zygomatic arch and is inserted in the outer surface of the ramus of the mandible. It also serves to elevate the mandible.

(The action of these muscles and the movement of the temporomandibular joint can be felt by placing the fingers in the appropriate positions at the side of the head while opening and closing the mouth and clenching the teeth.)

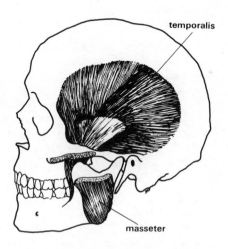

Fig. 2/14 Superficial muscles of mastication

Medial pterygoid. This is a thick quadrilateral muscle with its origin in the medial surface of the pterygoid plate of the sphenoid and its insertion in the lower part of the internal surface of the ramus of the mandible. Its action is to elevate the mandible and also to protrude the chin.

Lateral pterygoid. This is a short cone-shaped muscle originating from the infratemporal surface of the greater wing of the sphenoid and the lateral surface of the pterygoid plate. Its insertion is the front of the neck of the condyle and the joint capsule and disc of the temporomandibular joint. Its purpose is to draw the condyle forwards and inwards for side-to-side chewing, to protrude the chin and also to assist in depressing the mandible (opening the jaws).

All four of these muscles of mastication are developed from the 1st branchial arch and receive their motor nerve supply from the mandibular division of the 5th trigeminal nerve.

Hyoid muscles. Apart from the lateral pterygoid, the muscles which depress the mandible are weak by comparison with the elevator muscles and are assisted by the force of gravity. They are associated with the *hyoid bone* which lies in the front of the neck below the mandible. The hyoid is acted upon by the *infrahyoid muscles* (to the sternum, etc.) and by the *suprahyoid muscles* – the *digastric, mylohyoid* (the muscular floor of the mouth), *geniohyoid* and *stylohyoid*, the first three of which have attachments to the internal surface of the

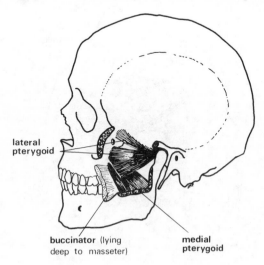

lateral
pterygoid

buccinator (lying
deep to masseter)

medial
pterygoid

Fig. 2/15 Deep muscles of mastication

body of the mandible. Their action in depressing the mandible may be further assisted by the superficial skin muscle of the neck, the *platysma*.

In summary, the possible movements of the mandible are: *protruding*; *elevating* to occlude the teeth; *retruding*; *depressing* to open the mouth, and *side to side* for chewing.

Mastication is also assisted by the actions of the *buccinator* muscle in the cheek and by the tongue.

The *buccinator* muscle of the wall of the cheek runs from the orbicularis oris in front to join the upper muscles of the pharynx at the *pterygomandibular raphe* which runs down from the region of the pterygoid plate to the mandible behind the third molar. Above and below, it arises from the outer surfaces of the alveolus opposite the molar teeth. It serves to press the cheek against the teeth and prevent food from collecting in the buccal *vestibule* (the oral space buccally and labially to the teeth) during mastication. This muscle is also used in blowing (*buccina* is Latin for a trumpet). Its motor nerve is the 7th or facial nerve.

Soft palate

The fold of tissue attached to the posterior border of the hard palate, which extends downwards and backwards and separates the nasal and oral parts of

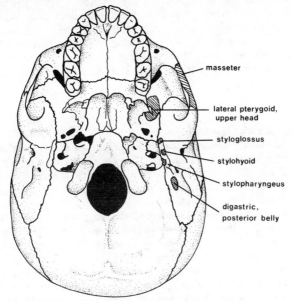

Fig. 2/16 Basal aspect of skull showing muscle attachments

the pharynx. It can be moved by muscles to seal off the nasal cavity, for example, during swallowing. The oral surface is covered with mucous membrane, and taste buds are present. The *uvula* is a small conical process extending from the mid-line of the free margin of the soft palate.

Tongue
This is a muscular organ associated with taste, swallowing and speech, and lies partly in the mouth and partly in the pharynx. The muscles of the root of the tongue are based on the hyoid bone and the genial tubercles of the mandible and other external muscles also join it from the styloid process, the palate and the pharynx. The motor nerve of the tongue muscles is the 12th or hypoglossal nerve.

The mucosa of the upper surface, sides and tip of the anterior two-thirds of the tongue is in the form of specialized *papillae: filiform* papillae, small, fine and thread-like; *fungiform* papillae, larger, round and deep red, and the *circumvallate* papillae which are eight to ten cup-shaped depressions in a V-shaped arrangement at the junction of the oral and pharyngeal parts of the tongue.

Taste buds are specialized nerve endings embedded in the papillae. The receptors sensitive to saltiness and sweetness lie mainly at the tip and front of the tongue, to sourness along the edges and to bitterness at the back of the tongue. The taste nerves for the anterior two-thirds are from the 7th facial nerve and the posterior third from the 9th glossopharyngeal nerve. (A further component of 'taste' is added by the smell of food carried to the olfactory nerve in the nose).

Muscles of facial expression
The facial muscles surround the openings of the eyes, nose, mouth and ears and serve as constrictors or dilators. They are all developed from the 2nd branchial arch and are served by its nerve, the 7th facial nerve. Their finely balanced action serves to change contours and express the emotions as in scowling, smiling, winking and so on.

The mouth is surrounded by a broad, flat ring of muscle, the *orbicularis oris*, and bands of muscle converge to join the angle of the mouth like the spokes of a wheel. The *zygomaticus* serves to raise, the *risorius* to draw back and the *depressor angularis* to lower the corner of the mouth in smiling or grinning or to turn the corner of the mouth down. Further groups of muscles attached to the mid-line of the lips (e.g. *levator labii superioris* in the upper, *mentalis* in the lower) serve to move these sections independently and to purse and pout the lips.

SALIVARY GLANDS

Parotid gland

This, the largest salivary gland, is wrapped around the posterior border of the ramus of the mandible and its associated structures. (It is the gland that commonly swells up in mumps.) It produces thin, serous saliva which is transmitted to the mouth through the parotid duct (*Stenson's duct*) which penetrates the buccinator muscle and opens opposite the second upper molar tooth.

Submandibular gland

This lies in the submandibular fossa on the inner surface of the body of the mandible and rests partially on the mylohyoid muscle. It produces a mucoserous saliva which is conducted forward through the submandibular duct (*Wharton's duct*) which opens at the *sublingual papilla* at one side of the *lingual fraenum* (the mid-line fold of mucosa beneath the tongue).

Sublingual gland

This is the smallest of the three main salivary glands and lies just beneath the mucosa of the floor of the mouth in the sublingual fossa of the body of the mandible. It produces a mainly thick, mucous saliva which passes straight into the mouth through some 10 to 20 sublingual ducts which open near the submandibular duct under the tongue.

The secretory, *secretomotor*, nerves for the salivary glands arise in the *salivatory centre* of the brain. They pass to the parotid gland via the 9th glossopharyngeal nerve, the tympanic branch fibres joining the *auriculotemporal nerve* which serves the area. The secretomotor nerves to the submandibular and sublingual glands are carried by a branch of the 7th facial nerve, the *chorda tympani*, via the *lingual nerve*.

Mucous glands

Those of the oral mucosa are numerous and all produce their addition to the saliva in the oral cavity.

In summary, the functions of saliva are: in *digestion* (it contains ptyalin); the *lubrication* of the food bolus; its *cleansing* action (removing food particles from the teeth); its *antibacterial* action used for protection, and its *buffer action* which stabilizes changes in the acid/alkali balance of the mouth.

NERVE SUPPLY OF THE TEETH AND ORAL TISSUES

The nerves supplying this region are the 5th trigeminal, the 7th facial, 9th glossopharyngeal and the 12th hypoglossal cranial nerves.

Note: Please refer to page 152 for the table of nerve supply to the individual teeth and surrounding structures (together with local anaesthesia used).

Trigeminal nerve (5th)

This is the largest cranial nerve. It is sensory for the face, scalp, mouth, teeth and nose, and motor to the muscles of mastication. It has a large sensory root and a smaller motor root and is divided into three main branches or divisions: the *ophthalmic*, the *maxillary* and the *mandibular*.

1. Ophthalmic nerve. This enters the orbit through the superior orbital fissure and divides into three branches, the *lacrimal, frontal* and *nasociliary* nerves. It is sensory to the eye, to the skin of the nose, forehead, eyelids and scalp and also part of the nasal mucosa. The frontal nerve passes through the *supraorbital notch*.

2. Maxillary nerve. This leaves the cranium through the *foramen rotundum*, crosses the *pterygopalatine fossa* and enters the orbit via the *inferior orbital fissure*. It then passes into the infraorbital groove and is transmitted through the infraorbital foramen to the surface of the cheek.

In the pterygopalatine fossa it gives off three branches:

The zygomatic nerve. This enters the zygomatic bone and sends branches to the temporal fossa and to the skin of the cheek via the zygomatic-facial foramen.

The ganglionic nerve. This supplies the *sphenopalatine ganglion*, which is linked with the facial nerve and sends branches mainly to the palate, nose and pharynx. The *greater palatine nerve* descends through the greater palatine foramen and runs forwards to serve the mucosa of the hard palate and adjacent gingivae. The *long sphenopalatine nerve* descends through the incisive fossa to serve the palatal mucosa behind the incisor teeth.

The posterior superior dental nerve. Branches from this nerve pass into the posterior surface of the maxilla to run in the canals in the wall of the sinus on their way to join the *middle superior dental* branches. Together they serve the lining of the sinus, the nearby molar and premolar teeth and their associated periodontal structures and cheek mucosa.

In the infraorbital canal the maxillary nerve gives off the *middle superior dental* and *anterior superior dental* branches. The former serves the upper teeth in communication with the posterior superior dental nerve branches. The anterior branch passes through a sinuous canal in the anterior wall of the sinus and its branches serve the incisor and canine teeth and the floor of the nasal cavity.

The maxillary nerve finally passes through the infraorbital foramen and gives off its terminal branches: *palpebral* to the lower eyelid, *nasal* to the nose and *labial* to the cheek, upper lip and local oral mucosa.

3. *Mandibular nerve.* The sensory root of this nerve is joined by the small motor root as it leaves the *foramen ovale* deep to the lateral pterygoid muscle.

The anterior trunk. This gives off motor branches to the muscles of mastication, the *medial pterygoid, lateral pterygoid, temporal* and *masseteric* nerves. It also gives off a sensory branch, the *buccal* nerve, which supplies the mucosa lining the cheek and the posterior buccal surface of the mandibular alveolar mucosa.

The posterior trunk. This divides into three branches: the *auriculotemporal* nerve which runs backwards behind the mandibular joint, communicates with the 7th facial nerve and serves the region of the ear, the joint, the parotid gland and the temporal skin, the *lingual* nerve which passes forwards to serve the mucous membrane of the anterior two-thirds of the tongue, the floor of the mouth and the lingual surface of the mandibular gingivae, and the *inferior dental* nerve. This gives off a small *mylohyoid* branch to the mylohyoid muscle and the anterior belly of the digastric muscle before it enters the mandibular foramen to run in the mandibular canal of the body of the mandible, giving off further branches to the molar and premolar teeth and their periodontal structures and associated buccal mucosa. At the mental foramen the *mental* nerve emerges to serve the skin and mucosa of the lip while the *incisive* nerve runs on in the bone to serve the incisor and canine teeth and their associated structures.

Facial nerve (7th)

This is the nerve of the second or hyoid arch and serves the muscles forming it including the muscles of the face, ear and scalp. Its terminal branches fan out from the borders of the parotid gland: the *postauricular*, the *temporal*, the *zygomatic*, the *buccal*, the *mandibular* and the *cervical*. The *chorda tympani* transmits secretomotor fibres on their way to the submandibular and sublingual glands and also carries taste sensory fibres from the anterior two-thirds of the tongue.

Glossopharyngeal nerve (9th)

This has sensory branches from the pharynx, tonsils and the posterior third of the tongue. It is secretomotor to the parotid gland and motor to the *stylopharyngeus*, a muscle of the pharynx.

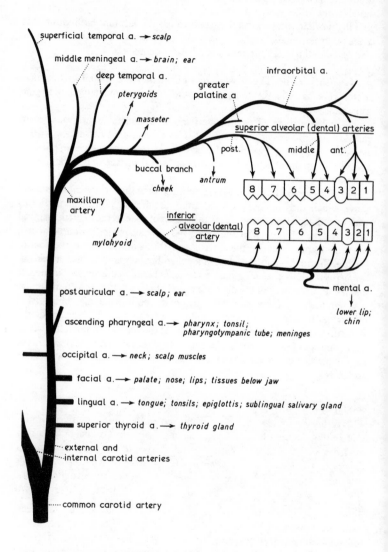

Fig. 2/17 Blood supply to the jaws, teeth and adjacent tissues

Hypoglossal nerve (12th)
This is the motor nerve of the tongue serving styloglossus, hyoglossus, geniohyoid, genioglossus muscles and the intrinsic muscle fibres of that organ.

BLOOD SUPPLY TO THE TEETH AND ORAL TISSUES
See Fig. 2/17.

The main arteries of the head and neck are the two *common carotid* arteries which divide into the *internal* and *external carotids* at the level of the thyroid cartilage of the larynx, the former going on to supply the inner parts of the cranium and orbit.

External carotid artery
This passes upwards through the neck giving off branches until it terminates at its final divisions within the structure of the parotid gland, level with the neck of the condyle. There are eight branches: the *superior thyroid, lingual, facial, occipital, ascending pharyngeal, posterior auricular, superficial temporal* and *maxillary* arteries.

The blood supply of the teeth is mainly from the lingual and maxillary arteries and most of their branches run on similar courses to the nerves, as also do the veins.

Lingual artery. This runs forward in a loop on the constrictor muscle of the pharynx in close association with the hypoglossal nerve at times and then rises to run on the inferior surface of the tongue near the mid-line, now accompanied by the lingual nerve. It serves the tongue and the floor of the mouth.

Maxillary artery. This arises deep to the neck of the condyle of the mandible and passes in relationship to the lateral pterygoid muscle on its way to the pterygomandibular fossa. Its first or mandibular part gives off branches to the ear and the brain (*meningeal* artery), before the *inferior dental* artery descends to the mandibular foramen, giving off the *mylohyoid* branch, and entering the mandibular canal to accompany the inferior dental nerve to serve the teeth and mental foramen region.

The second or pterygoid part of the maxillary artery has *temporal, pterygoid, masseteric* and *buccal* branches which closely follow the similar branches of the mandibular nerve to their muscles.

The third or pterygopalatine part has several more branches of dental importance. Branches of the *posterior superior dental* artery enter the posterior surface of the maxilla and serve the lining of the antrum, the premolar and molar teeth and the alveolar process. The *infraorbital* artery has branches to the incisor and canine region. The *greater palatine* and *sphenopalatine* arteries descend through the greater palatine foramen and incisive fossa of the maxilla to serve the palatal mucosa.

Facial artery. This supplies tissues which include the muscles of facial expression, the sublingual gland, the soft palate and tonsil area and is of special dental interest because it supplies the labial arteries to the lips.

CHAPTER THREE

Bacteriology and Pathology

Bacteriology is the science which deals with micro-organisms and pathology is the study of diseases and their effects on the functions of the body.

BACTERIOLOGY

Bacteria
See Fig. 3/1.
These are microscopic, single-celled organisms that are classified at the lower limit of the scale of living things. In favourable conditions they multiply by simple cell division. There are many different species of bacteria and they can be identified in the laboratory because of their different sizes and shapes, by the way they grow in colonies on special nutrient materials (culture media) and in the way they can be stained with special dye solutions.

Viruses
A virus is an extremely minute body often several hundred times smaller than a bacterium and thus invisible under the most powerful optical microscope and able to pass easily through the finest bacteria-stopping filters. They multiply inside the cells of the infected host. Rabies, herpes and the common cold are all examples of diseases caused by viruses.

Fungi
These are simple plants which lack chlorophyll and are either saprophytes or parasites. Examples include yeasts, moulds and mushrooms. Some fungi can cause diseases in man.

Saprophytes and parasites
Bacteria are found to be widely distributed in nature for they exist in vast numbers in soil, water, air and in all decaying organic matter. Those called collectively *saprophytes* exist on dead material, while *parasites* grow on living tissues. Some bacteria can adapt to exist in both situations. Like plants they will grow faster in ideal conditions. Each organism may then divide every 20 minutes and thus one cell could produce many millions in the course of a

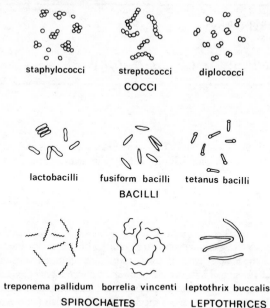

staphylococci streptococci diplococci

COCCI

lactobacilli fusiform bacilli tetanus bacilli

BACILLI

treponema pallidum borrelia vincenti leptothrix buccalis

SPIROCHAETES LEPTOTHRICES

Fig. 3/1 Bacterial types

single day. Variations of temperature, oxygen level, available food and moisture will all affect this phenomenal growth rate. When very unfavourable conditions arise some bacteria, such as the tetanus bacillus (the organism that causes tetanus or 'lockjaw'), can form *spores* which are tiny seed-like granules surrounded by a dense protective capsule. These spores can survive in boiling water (100 °C) for almost an hour and still be capable of commencing new growth when they reach favourable conditions once more.

Pathogens

Only a small group of bacteria are able to cause disease in man and these are called *pathogens*. Pathogenic organisms produce powerful poisons called *toxins* which can give rise to the symptoms of the disease. *Endotoxins* tend to affect the tissues near to the infecting source and may be produced by the body of the organism itself after it has died. *Exotoxins*, on the other hand, can affect parts of the body that are some distance away from the site of the originating bacteria; for example, in diphtheria the infecting organisms remain in the nasopharynx, but the exotoxins, getting into the circulation, can cause heart failure or nervous paralysis of the limbs. Common *pyogenic* (pus-forming) wound infections are caused by such organisms as staphylococcus and streptococcus.

Staphylococci. These are spherical bodies of about 1 micron (μ) (0.001mm) in diameter which divide in every plane and are thus arranged typically in grape-like clusters. Three types are known: *Staphylococcus aureus*, *Staphylococcus albus* and *Staphylococcus citreus*, so named because they produce golden, white and lemon-yellow colonies respectively when grown in the laboratory. *Staphylococcus aureus* is the most virulent and is responsible for boils, skin abscesses and other superficial infections. If it manages to spread to deeper tissues or enter the blood-stream it can cause such things as bone marrow infection (osteomyelitis) or generalized blood infection (septicaemia).

Streptococci. These are also spherical bodies of a similar size, but as they divide repeatedly in the same plane they are arranged characteristically in chains, like beads on a string. They can be subclassified as haemolytic, non-haemolytic or viridans because of their varying ability to dissolve red blood cells in a special laboratory culture medium. *Streptococcus haemolyticus* is present in the nose and throat of many people and is a potential source of infection to themselves as well as the other people with whom they come in contact. This is one of the reasons why surgeons wear masks when operating. This organism can infect wounds and cause abscesses or it may give rise to more spreading and generalized infections as in scarlet fever, pneumonia or middle ear infections. Of particular interest is *Streptococcus viridans* for it may be found in dental abscesses and is thought to have a link with certain kinds of infection of the inner surface of the heart and its valves (bacterial endocarditis). Non-haemolytic streptococci give rise to infections similar but less severe than those caused by the other classes.

PATHOLOGY

Protective mechanisms of the body

Countless numbers of bacteria live normally on the human body surfaces: on the skin, in the hair, in the mouth, nose and throat. They are constantly present in the air that is breathed in and in all food that is eaten. Several species of organisms are in permanent residence in the intestines and some even manufacture valuable nutritive materials for the body. Most of these organisms would cause infection and disease if they were able to penetrate the body's defensive system.

The human body has several protective barriers and mechanisms to resist invasion by pathogenic organisms. An intact skin and to a lesser extent an intact mucous membrane will shield the body against most bacteria. In addition sweat and other skin secretions all tend to wash away and discourage the growth of organisms. Tears, nasal secretions and saliva also have this constant cleaning action and many of these surface secretions contain a substance, lysozyme, which has a strong bactericidal effect. The gastric juices are strongly acid and capable of destroying most bacteria ingested in food. The lungs and respiratory tract are coated with a layer of sticky mucus which is constantly being moved, by specialized epithelial cells, against the incoming breath and thus carries any potential irritant or infection back to the throat where it is swallowed and dealt with by the gastric juices.

Immunity. This is a term used to describe an individual's general bodily resistance to infection. This may be *natural immunity* where a species, race or individual is resistant to a particular pathogen (for example, man does not catch distemper from a dog) or it may be an *acquired immunity* as when recovery from a single attack of a disease gives lifelong protection from a second attack (such as diphtheria, measles) by the production of *antibodies* in the blood.

Vaccines and other products can be designed to produce special protection against certain diseases, such as hepatitis and tetanus. Weakened and inactivated organisms or extracts of the infective agent are injected subcutaneously (under the skin) to stimulate active immunity without the subject having to suffer the disease.

Infection
Infection occurs when there is a successful invasion of the body by living pathogenic organisms with consequent damage to the host. The infecting organism can be transmitted to a human being in several ways:

1. By direct or indirect contact
2. By droplets or airborne infection
3. By being swallowed
4. By an insect or animal contact.

An organism's capacity to overcome the body's defences and invade the host depends upon its virulence, the power of the toxins it can produce, the numbers of bacteria that are present at the point of infection and the exact portal of entry. The host defences will be able to protect a small, shallow scratch more easily than a deep, jagged wound or an extensive burn.

Acute inflammation
This is the rapid reaction of the tissues to an irritant (bacterial, chemical, physical) which causes an injury that is not severe enough to kill them. Chemicals from the damaged cells go into the circulation and cause an urgent local, and later a general alarm reaction. The small blood vessels and capillaries adjacent to the wound become dilated and make the surrounding

skin and tissues red and hot, then fluid and cells exude from these dilated vessels and swelling occurs. The sensory nerves to the area are stimulated by the toxins and the increasing pressure of the inflammatory exudate and give the sensation of throbbing pain. The structures and organs in the region all suffer an impairment of function.

Thus the cardinal signs and symptoms of acute inflammation are:

1. Heat
2. Redness
3. Swelling
4. Pain
5. Loss of function.

By this process fluids, specialized blood cells and complex chemical agents are brought to the area to localize and counteract the effects of the injury and attempt to resist infection and kill any invading organisms. The most important role in this cellular defence is played by the white cells (leucocytes) of blood, particularly the polymorphonuclear leucocytes which can move independently through the body tissues and actually engulf or 'eat' a dozen or more invading organisms and thus imprison and kill them. Masses of these white cells are attracted to an inflamed region. The products of this battle between the cells and organisms are gradually washed into the drainage system of the lymphatics and passed on to the nearest *lymphatic glands*. These glands may soon swell as a result of their increased activity.

The general bodily effects of the onset of acute inflammation are usually a feeling of chill and an attack of shivering, followed by a rise in temperature to above 37.2°C, with an associated rise in the pulse rate and a general sensation of illness. Thus the body physically aids the defensive mechanisms by increasing the speed of the general circulation and the passage of blood to the damaged part, by making the inflamed region painful and difficult to use so that it is rested and helped to recover, and by making the host feel unwell and less inclined to squander his general strength. At the same time the rise in body temperature helps to increase general cellular activity.

Acute inflammation is generally only of short duration and can proceed to one of several conclusions:

1. It can successfully overcome the infection and the inflamed part is then repaired or replaced with scar tissue.
2. It can result in the formation of pus (suppuration).
3. It can extend, as when the organisms overcome the host's defences, and the infection passes more deeply into the body involving tissue spaces, structures and organs and perhaps invading the bloodstream.
4. It can become *chronic* and persistent.

5. The tissue may die (*necrosis*: death of a small number of cells; *gangrene*: death of a large number of cells, such as a finger or a limb).

Suppuration. This occurs if the bacteria are able to kill some of the host's cells in the infected part. This inflammatory exudate is then full of living, dead and degenerating white cells together with living and dead organisms and tissue cells and the resultant thick, creamy, opaque and sometimes bloodstained material is called *pus*.

Abscesses. An abscess is a collection of pus confined within the walls of a cavity formed by tissue degeneration. The essential local treatment of an abscess is to open it up to the surface and thus allow adequate drainage of the pus. This is achieved, for instance, in an apical dental abscess by opening the root canal or removing the infected tooth. When a deep abscess bursts through the overlying tissues to drain spontaneously on to the surface, the opening is called a *sinus*, for example, the discharging sinus over the apex of a chronically infected tooth.

The general treatment of inflammation is aimed at maintaining the patient's strength, general health and resistance and reinforcing these when necessary with carefully chosen antibiotic drugs, such as penicillin, to which the causative organisms are known to be sensitive.

Cysts. A cyst is an abnormal cavity or sac within the body lined by well-defined epithelial and fibrous tissue and filled with a fluid or semisolid material. Dental cysts are usually formed from a small cluster of epithelial cells deeply embedded in the tissues. As these cells multiply into a clump, the cells in the centre become deprived of nutrition from the surrounding blood supply and they degenerate and liquefy, while those at the outside continue to survive and multiply. Fluid pressure increases inside the cavity as the products build up inside the wall of cells and a balloon-like expansion takes place.

Tumours. A tumour is a swelling, usually due to a new growth of cells (*neoplasm*) arising without known cause and growing without any relationship to normal growth, repair or health and thus serving no useful purpose. Tumours may be *benign* (localized and not invasive) or *malignant* (progressively invasive and growing at the expense of local tissue). Primarily malignant tumours can give rise to secondary 'seedling' tumours in other parts of the body when tiny fragments of the original tumour are carried in the lymphatics or bloodstream to other tissues or organs and start to grow there.

Ulcers. An ulcer is a localized lesion of the skin or mucous membrane where destruction of the surface epithelium exposes the deeper tissues in an open sore which may become secondarily infected. Ulcers may occur in the mouth that are due to a variety of causes, for example malignant changes, traumatic ulcers due to scratches or ill-fitting dentures, or herpetic ulcers due to a virus infection, etc. Ulcers require urgent examination, diagnosis and treatment.

Diagnostic aids
Laboratory investigations for a patient are often an important aid to diagnosis and treatment planning. The taking, handling and transport of all these samples for diagnosis have to be carried out under strictly controlled aseptic conditions. This is (1) to protect the specimen and (2) to ensure that there is no danger of cross-infection.

Swabs. A swab can be taken of pus from an infected surface and then laboratory tests may be carried out to identify the pathogenic organisms and discover the drugs to which it is sensitive so that appropriate treatment can be started.

Blood tests. A blood test can reveal important details about a patient such as his bleeding and clotting times, the number and type of blood cells present, the haemoglobin level, the blood group, the presence of infecting organisms and so on, as well as helping in the detection of specific diseases.

Biopsies. For a biopsy a small piece of diseased tissue is cut out of the lesion under examination and is then prepared, sectioned, stained and studied under the microscope. After this a detailed report can be made about the condition of the tissue and cells of the affected part.

DENTAL PATHOLOGY

Dental caries
See Fig. 3/2.
This disease is a localized, post-eruptive, pathological process of external origin involving the softening and disintegration of the hard tooth tissues and proceeding to the formation of a cavity. It is the most universally prevalent disease afflicting the human race and is found particularly in people who live in civilized communities and eat a highly refined diet. The developmental pits and fissures are the first parts of the teeth to be affected and then the interproximal contact areas. In middle age, the necks of the teeth are more commonly at risk as the gingivae recede. At all stages local loss of tooth structure will allow the stagnation of food debris and possibly food packing between the teeth and damage to the gingival and periodontal structures.

Several theories have been put forward to explain the mechanisms

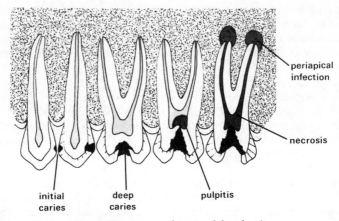

Fig. 3/2 The progress of untreated dental caries

responsible for the production of dental caries and the disease is the subject of constant research.

The most popular theory suggests that caries is due to the attack of acid-producing bacteria. Organisms can be found on the surfaces of the teeth having the ability to convert sugars and other fermentable carbohydrates to lactic and other acids. When these organisms are allowed to collect undisturbed on the tooth surface, together with deposits of mucin from the saliva, epithelial cells and food debris, they quickly form a strongly adherent film called *dental plaque*. This deposit will occur most easily in areas that are not self-cleansing, for example, pits and fissures and interdental spaces. These large numbers of organisms, protected from the acid-neutralizing or buffering effects of saliva, can rapidly convert the sugary food debris and produce an acid strong enough to attack the enamel, and they will receive further supplies of sugars and fermentable carbohydrate in each mouthful that is put into the mouth. Gradually the surface of the enamel is decalcified and takes on a whitish, chalky appearance before it disintegrates allowing the organisms to invade the tooth. When the full depth of the enamel is involved, the process crosses the enamel–dentine (amelodentinal) junction and the inorganic part of the dentine is attacked and decalcified. This softened dentine, now directly open to the mouth, is soon invaded by protein-dissolving (proteolytic) organisms and the cavity rapidly enlarges, partly by extension along the enamel–dentine junction and partly by deeper penetration along the dentinal tubules towards the pulp. The pulp reacts by trying to wall off the approaching process by forming secondary dentine within the pulp chamber. Unless the carious process is arrested the pulp becomes inflamed and painful. Without treatment the pulp eventually dies, with relief of the pain, and the bacteria can then invade the pulp chamber. The infection may then pass through the apical foramen of the tooth and cause a periapical abscess. An acute periapical abscess causes pain and swelling of the alveolus ('gumboil') or of the facial tissues and lymph nodes in the region.

Occult (or hidden) *caries* can occur occasionally when the organisms gain access to the dentine via a fine, almost undetectable tract through the enamel (which in this case does not disintegrate) and the carious process mushrooms into the dentine. It has been suggested that this may be due to fluoride-strengthened enamel that does not collapse easily when undermined.

Periodontal disease
See Fig. 3/3.
This is the general term used to describe abnormalities of the periodontium or supporting structures of the teeth (the cementum, the periodontal membrane, the alveolar bone and the overlying and investing tissues).

Inflammation of the gingival tissues (gingivitis) may arise from a variety of causes. The commonest local causes include soft foods that do nothing to stimulate and harden the gingival tissues; sharp, hard foods that scratch and damage the gingival tissues; inefficient tooth brushing and food debris stagnation; irregularly arranged teeth and traumatic bites; untreated dental caries or inadequate and badly contoured restorations; ill-fitting partial dentures or orthodontic appliances; and the drying due to mouth breathing. Gingivitis is often associated with the formation of tartar (calculus) on the

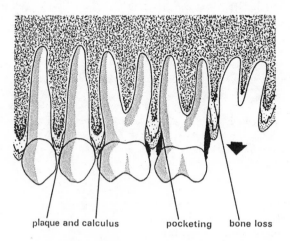

plaque and calculus   pocketing   bone loss

Fig. 3/3 The progress of untreated periodontal disease

teeth. There may also be general factors involved such as vitamin deficiencies, blood disorders and drugs.

In chronic marginal gingivitis the gum margins are very slightly swollen and may bleed easily. If the disease is neglected and inflammation spreads deeper to involve the periodontal membrane, the gingivae become detached from the necks of the teeth and a pocket is formed in which further food debris and inflammatory products accumulate. This serious condition is usually painless and may pass unnoticed by the patient.

Gradually, if still untreated, the gingival attachment recedes towards the apical region of the tooth, the pockets enlarge, the fibres of the periodontal membrane are progressively destroyed, the gingivae recede, the alveolar bone of the socket is resorbed and the tooth loosens.

Delay in discovering and treating this slow, insidious disease process will lead to the loss of many teeth, particularly in the over-35 age group, although the first stages of the disease can often be detected in adolescence.

CHAPTER FOUR

Practice Organization

The majority of dental surgery assistants (DSAs) are employed in general practice, although they may also work in other clinical situations such as dental clinics, dental hospitals, dental departments of general hospitals and in specialist practices.

While this chapter describes in outline how the duties of the DSA fit into the organization of general practice, it must be remembered that each individual practice has its own characteristics shaped by its situation and patients, size and internal layout and the dental surgeon's own personality and requirements.

The DSA must keep a flexible attitude of mind when she starts a new job in practice and be willing to learn about unfamiliar routines and working conditions before presuming to contribute suggestions based upon her own knowledge and experience.

The DSA becomes a key member of the dental health team, headed by the dental surgeon, which is devoted to the smooth, efficient running of the practice and to providing the highest standard of dental care for the patients. In small practices the DSA may be the only assistant the dental surgeon requires, but in large practices there will be more than one DSA and possibly a dental technician, a secretary/receptionist and an oral hygienist on the staff.

It is most important that the DSA maintains a professional relationship at all times with the patients, the dental surgeon and the other members of the dental team. She must not gossip about the privileged information she will gain within the practice; she must devote all her attention to the work of the practice while on duty; personal matters should be set aside to be dealt with outside surgery hours, for example, the telephone must not be used for personal calls. Everything must be done to shield the dental surgeon from all unnecessary distractions so that he may concentrate all his time and attention upon the central and prime purpose of caring for his patients. In addition, skilled chairside assistance will mean that he will be able to work faster and more efficiently, thus making a greater contribution to the health of the community, as well as earning more money for the practice.

The rooms in general dental practice are usually allocated to serve different purposes as shown in Fig. 4/1. In some practices a room can have more than one function, for example, office/staff room or office/waiting room, while others may not have a laboratory or a dark room.

The duties of the trained DSA will include reception, surgery and secretarial work. Although in larger practices these duties may be shared between several members of the staff, the DSA must be capable of undertaking all these duties if required to do so.

RECEPTION

One of the most important aspects of a successful dental practice is the atmosphere surrounding the reception of patients and other callers on the telephone and at the door. This, the first contact that the perhaps nervous and apprehensive patient makes with the practice will immediately set the the tone of the whole encounter because it will be presumed to reflect the general interest and attitude of mind of the whole team.

Telephone technique

1. All incoming calls should be answered as soon as possible.
2. Always smile while you speak on the telephone for this will give your voice a friendly, pleasant sound. You can remind yourself to smile by having a mirror in front of the telephone.
3. Answer the telephone efficiently by giving your own number and perhaps adding 'Mr Tooth's dental surgery – can I help you?' If you are very busy never say 'Hold on a minute!' and put down the receiver. Instead, ask the caller if he is prepared to wait or if he could call back in a few minutes, otherwise note the telephone number and arrange to call back later yourself.
4. Keep calls brief and to the point. Other patients may want to contact the practice also.
5. Take down any messages accurately and make sure that they reach their destination quickly. A message pad and pencil are essential next to the telephone.

Note: Some practices have complicated telephone systems and answering machines. Make sure that you understand fully how to use unfamiliar equipment.

Appointment book

The appointment book rules the speed at which a practice runs and the dental surgeon will indicate how much time he requires for each patient. Keep the book entries in pencil for easy alteration. Write in all appointments at the moment that they are made and always give the patient a written

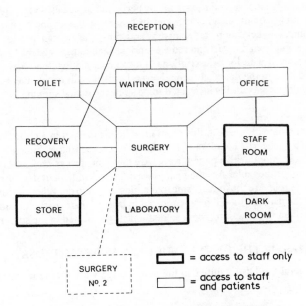

Fig. 4/1 Layout of rooms in a general dental practice

appointment card. Do not book long appointments so that they will overlap the lunch break.

General reception
When patients arrive they are usually met by a member of the team and conducted to the waiting room. Make sure that everything is done to soothe their senses of sight, hearing and smell which may be enhanced by nervousness. All the rooms pertaining to the practice must be kept clean, bright and pleasant. All offensive odours including tobacco, the staff's lunchtime snacks, strong antiseptics, etc. should be banned or dealt with by an aerosol air freshener.

The DSA must always have a neat, clean and tidy appearance, with a clean uniform, unobtrusive make-up and a neat hairstyle. Obviously she has well-cared-for teeth and good oral hygiene. She must balance speed and efficiency with professional charm, cheerfulness and sympathy when she greets a patient. Speed does not mean running about – 'a nurse only runs in the event of fire or haemorrhage'. She must remember that what for her is just another routine visit to the practice may represent a long-dreaded, major event from the patient's point of view. People under stress may react in quite uncharacteristic ways, for example, by becoming more talkative or quick to take offence or, at the other extreme, by becoming quieter and even tearful. Smiling, low-key, interested sympathy and 'time to listen' can help to soothe the patient from the start and reduce tensions in the surgery later. Try not to get involved with long descriptions of symptoms that will only have to be retold later to the dental surgeon. Never discuss details of treatment at this stage unless specifically instructed to do so by the dental surgeon.

Waiting room

In common with the rest, this room must be maintained in a clean, bright, warm and cheerful condition. Sit in the waiting room yourself now and then and look around with a patient's eye. Are the chair springs broken? Is there dust under the table? Are the magazines dogeared and out of date? Are the ashtrays full? Are the mirrors smeared or dusty? and so on. Where security is good the patients should be encouraged to take off their coats and hats and leave them in the waiting room so that time is not wasted in the surgery.

DUTIES OF THE DENTAL SURGERY ASSISTANT (DSA)

In general the DSA's duties in the dental surgery are concerned with the following.

Maintenance of equipment

The equipment, instruments and furnishings must be maintained in good working order and in a high state of cleanliness and preparation. This can be done efficiently if special checklists are made out to indicate a schedule of daily, weekly, monthly and half-yearly tasks which will include everything from switching the equipment on in the morning, oiling the handpieces, cleaning out the spittoon traps, draining the air compressor, polishing and cleaning the surfaces in the surgery right through to arranging a regular visit by the maintenance engineer from the dental company's service department. Checklists mean that you do not have to rely on your memory.

Expendable items

The DSA must ensure that adequate stocks of expendable drugs, materials and instruments are immediately available. Make frequent stock list checks with your dental surgeon. Always keep available a spare operating light bulb and fuses for the dental unit. Know where tools such as a screwdriver are kept.

Patients' records

All the relevant dental records, radiographs, appliances and models must be immediately available for all patients visiting the surgery on that day. This usually means that they have to be got out of the files the day before. It is helpful to keep a list of the day's appointments in the surgery and at reception.

Preparation of patients for treatment

The DSA must assist patients into the surgery and get them settled in the chair and prepared for treatment with the minimum of delay; for example, ladies should be given a tissue to remove their lipstick.

Assistance during treatment

The DSA must produce instruments and materials as necessary during treatment, quickly and efficiently and to assist the dental surgeon as he requests it. The extent to which the DSA is expected to help in this respect will vary from one dental surgeon to another and will depend also upon the design of the surgery. It usually involves suction, retraction, manipulation of the air and water syringes, changing burs in the handpiece, passing instruments and mixing and passing materials. The DSA acts as a witness to treatment and also as a chaperon.

Making the next appointment

The DSA must assist the patient from the surgery without unnecessary delay and arrange for the next appointment to be made or for the patient's name to be placed in the recall file.

Treatment record

An adequate written record must be kept of all treatment provided.

Cleaning up

The DSA must tidy up between patients, clean and sterilize the instruments and remove all traces of the visit.

Awareness of special patient problems

Although every patient attending the dental surgery must be granted full attention and care at all times, certain categories of patient present special problems that require extra thought and preparation. These are usually patients suffering from a particular disability or handicap. Such disabilities are commonly classified as follows: *medical*, for example, the asthmatic patient or the patient who is recovering from a heart condition and taking drugs to prevent further blood clots occurring; *physical*, for example, the blind or paralysed patient; *mental*, for example, the patient with Down's syndrome (mongolism), or the retarded patient; and *social*, for example, the child from a broken home. The extent of special care for such patients may even require the dental surgeon and the DSA to make a domiciliary visit to carry out dental treatment in the patient's own home.

SURGERY DESIGN

There are many different working arrangements but they generally fall into one of the following categories:

The dental surgeon works standing up. All equipment and cabinets are fixed, but within easy reach a step or two away from the chair. A single dental unit will suffice. The DSA assists from the patient's left side when required. This arrangement is now only used for certain aspects of dental treatment, for example, for the extraction of teeth.

The dental surgeon is seated. This means that he is no longer mobile and all equipment has to be brought nearer to the chair for him to reach it, or else handed to him. The DSA must spend more time at the chairside, but will have to have access to equipment on both sides of the chair during treatment.

Four-handed dentistry. The dental surgeon and the DSA are both seated. All equipment is within easy reach of both of them, or the DSA only, and can be passed freely to and fro. This is a less tiring arrangement and means that four hands are available to carry out treatment in the patient's mouth. It may take a few weeks for the close support teamwork required to be achieved but once gained, the speed of treatment to a high standard is greatly enhanced. Low-level stools will require low-level working surfaces and a dental chair without too many levers, etc. projecting in the way of the team's knees. The DSA may move away from the chairside for other duties such as sterilizing instruments.

Six-handed dentistry. The dental surgeon and the DSA are both seated as before, but to minimize their time away from the chairside, a second DSA is always available to sterilize and replenish instruments, prepare materials and generally work in support of the other two. There should be frequent interchange of the two DSAs to ensure that they are both fully trained in chairside duties and thus avoid the dental surgeon becoming totally dependent on one assistant with unsettling results to the practice in the event of holidays, illness and so on.

Surgery equipment
The following items will be found in most dental surgeries:

A dental unit. This contains and supports such things as the operating light, air-spray, water-spray, suction and saliva ejector, the dental engine, air-rotor or air-motor, a spittoon and a sterilizable working surface or bracket table. The unit may be a single pedestal or split into two sections one on each side of the chair.

A dental chair. Most dental surgeons now operate with the patient lying in the supine position, and it is important to protect the patient's airway and eyes. High-speed suction facilities are essential. The dental chair has a mechanism (sometimes programmed) for raising, lowering and tilting it until the patient's mouth is at a convenient working height for the dental surgeon. In some circumstances the patient has to be treated sitting up, for example, if suffering from an arthritic condition, and most modern dental chairs can be adjusted to accommodate these requirements.

Cabinets and trolleys. These are best grouped as close as possible to the working area so that instruments, materials and working surfaces are conveniently to hand during treatment procedures.

Operating stools. When the dental team can sit down to work they will be less tired at the end of the day. Positioning is very important, otherwise the DSA may get into the bad habit of working in a crouched, unbalanced position that can be just as tiring as working standing up. Try to sit upright with both feet comfortably flat on the floor and the spine and neck straight and upright. Working surfaces and the patient's mouth height should ideally be at elbow height so that the hands and forearms are working in the least tiring position.

Sterilizing apparatus. Unless a sterile package or tray system is used, this apparatus must be switched on at the earliest opportunity in the day so that it is fully heated up and ready for action at the start of the treatment session.

X-ray apparatus. This generally requires little attention apart from cleaning and dusting the outer surfaces. The apparatus should be switched off at the main electric source when not in use. (Keep a careful eye on the condition of the exposed wiring, for these machines develop high voltages.)

Hand instruments. These must be maintained at a very high standard and checked frequently. Moving parts must be oiled regularly, for example, handpieces. The method of sharpening chisels and excavators can only be learned by watching a practical demonstration. They can be ruined by inexpert grinding and some dental surgeons prefer to sharpen hand instruments themselves.

Dental materials. These form an expensive item in any practice budget and should be used economically. Although replacement stocks must be available it is obviously ill-advised to order large quantities of materials which may deteriorate before they are used. Under normal conditions the DSA will not be expected to order any stocks without first consulting the dental surgeon about it.

The scrap residues of certain materials such as amalgam, mercury, gold and the lead foil from x-ray packages are valuable and should be saved up as they are saleable.

Some disposable items may be dangerous if they fall into wrong hands. The remains of drugs should be washed away down the sink. Infected and sharp items must be disposed of with great care. (See Chapter 5, Sterilization and prevention of cross-infection.)

Specialist apparatus. There may be many other pieces of apparatus present in the surgery, anaesthetic machines, spot-welders, ultrasonic scalers and so on, that will require special care and maintenance. The DSA should find out what unfamiliar apparatus is for, how it works and whether she is responsible for its maintenance. Some types of specialist apparatus are easily and expensively damaged by the untaught.

Emergency equipment. Make sure that you know where the surgical emergency equipment is kept and that it is always in good order. If any part of it is used at any time make sure that it is replaced immediately. See also Recovery Room below.

THE RECOVERY ROOM

This is used for patients who need to lie down for a while to recover from a general anaesthetic or from a reaction to treatment, such as fainting, before they are fit to leave for home.

Equipment
The equipment in a recovery room will usually consist of:

1. A firm couch and pillows with washable covers
2. A supply of blankets
3. A good light source at the patient's head for observing his colour and to illuminate any intraoral procedures
4. Bowls for vomit, blood and mouthwashing
5. A supply of towels, preferably disposable
6. Mouthwash cups
7. A mirror for the patients to tidy their appearance afterwards.

Emergency equipment
Emergency equipment and services may be duplicated here and in the surgery, for example, suction, oxygen, gags, airways, cardiac and respiratory

stimulant drugs, syringes and hypodermic needles, sterile artery forceps, gauze packs. In general practice this room may only be used at infrequent intervals, but it must be maintained in constant readiness and its contents and cleanliness should be added to the weekly checklist apart from the immediate cleaning that is required each time it is used.

DARK ROOM

This is where dental radiographs are processed and is used on all occasions when light-sensitive film has to be handled.

Essential features
These are:

1. Light-proof window covers
2. Photographic safe-lights and independent ordinary lights
3. A door-locking system so designed that there is no danger of accidental admission of light during film processing
4. Developing, washing and fixing tanks and a source of running water
5. Electric tank heaters and and thermometer
6. A clock with an alarm timing system
7. X-ray film hangers, films, cassettes and a store of chemicals
8. A place to hang processed films to dry
9. A container for scrap foil and a bin for waste paper
10. An adequate ventilation system to eliminate chemical fumes.

This room has to be kept clean and dust-free. Splashes of chemical solutions must be wiped up immediately. All solutions must be maintained as indicated in the manufacturers' instructions. *Note:* X-ray films can also be processed in daylight using special light-proof developing tanks and apparatus such as the Kodak 'Dentech' processor.

DENTAL LABORATORY

This is rarely in the DSA's province, but she needs to know where things are kept, particularly impressions, models and completed work. The liaison between the DSA and the laboratory technicians must be maintained at a friendly, mutually helpful level so that the work flows smoothly and adequate time is given for each laboratory stage to be completed. In all cases requiring laboratory work always consult the technician before arranging the patient's next appointment. Make sure that the work-slip is clearly made out. Ensure that cross-infection precautions are preserved between the surgery and the laboratory. If possible arrange for the work to be ready at the start of the morning or afternoon session so that the dental surgeon has time to examine it before the patient arrives. In some practices work is sent out to a laboratory and great care must be taken to pack fragile models and wax-ups with plenty of padding so that they are not damaged in transit. Some dental surgeons will teach their DSA to cast up impressions as soon as they are taken to avoid possible distortion or breakages if casting is delayed.

OFFICE

The DSA's duties and responsibilities in the office will vary from practice to practice. In some cases a special secretary is employed to run the office, while in other, smaller practices the DSA will be expected to carry out most of this work herself, under the supervision of the dental surgeon. The following lists briefly indicate some of the more important aspects of office work, but must not be regarded as comprehensive. The range of work may seem formidable, but it can be reduced to an easily controllable amount by a tidy, systematic approach. The future of office administration will obviously be affected by the rapidly expanding usage of microprocessors in the handling of information both in the form of figures and words and it may be assumed that the DSA will shortly be involved in this (Fig. 4/2).

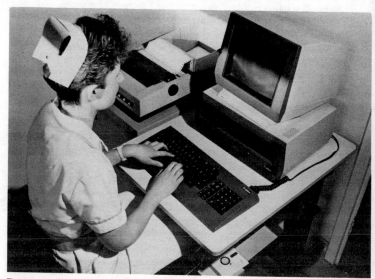

Fig. 4/2 A microprocessor system that can be used to handle information and records in dental practice

Current office computer set-ups consist basically of a keyboard, similar to that of a typewriter, a visual display unit (VDU) resembling a standard television screen, together with methods of electronically recording information on discs or tapes and a printout mechanism which itself can type like a typewriter. The computer can be used as a word processor. It can also store items such as address lists, details of patients' treatments, waiting lists, recall lists, stock control, accounting and tax details, and can recall and display or print out such information instantly. The data can be updated easily and the storage space required is much less than that for similar information on paper. The future uses of such apparatus appear to be limitless.

Office equipment

Desk or work table
Chairs
Good light source
Filing cabinets or cupboards, safe
  or cash box
Telephone

Typewriter
Computer/word processor
Computer disc files
Wastepaper basket
General reference books

Office stocks

Headed notepaper
Plain typing paper, top and copy
  qualities
Envelopes
Treatment record cards for new
  patients: both NHS and private
X-ray envelopes
NHS forms, envelopes, etc.
Anaesthetic consent forms
Bill forms
Receipt forms or book
Appointment cards

Recall cards
Laboratory slips
Message slips
Message pads
Carbon paper
Computer supplies: discs, printer
  ribbons, printout paper
Spare typewriter ribbon
Writing materials: pens, pencils,
  erasers, paper clips, etc.
Postage stamps
Dental health literature

Professional records

Patients' records and radiographs, filed as follows:
  NHS
  Private

On treatment
Off treatment
Awaiting payment
Patients' correspondence – doctors, dental surgeons, hospitals, NHS, etc.
Appointment book
Day book (records the fee earned immediately each patient leaves the surgery)
Models (under 200 models can be stored alphabetically, over 200 should be stored numerically and an index book used)

Recall system
Create a file with monthly divisions. Put the patient's name under the month you have promised to send a recall appointment. Review and act a month in advance.

Financial records
General accounts:
General account book
Petty cash book
Wages book
Bills and receipts of practice expenses
Patients' accounts:
Accounts for treatment completed/dates presented and paid
Day book, as mentioned above
Banking matters:
Bank statements, paying-in book, the practice cheque book
All these records have to be produced for the accountant annually for him to prepare a general statement of the affairs of the practice and deal with taxation matters
Tax matters:
Demands, letters, receipts
Postage book (records of postage stamps used and posting dates)

General information
Surgery routine check lists
Information book, which lists such things as the names, addresses and telephone numbers of: accountant; anaesthetist; electrician; equipment servicing agents; dental companies; plumber; special dental laboratories; laundry; printers, and so on
Stores lists with dates orders made and received
Drug lists
Poisons records
Accident record book

Precious metals record
Laundry book or lists
Practice documents:
  Instruction leaflets
  Hire purchase agreements
  Insurance policies, etc.
Holiday lists
Records of instruments being repaired or taken out of the practice for use
  elsewhere, for example, in an operating theatre

CHAPTER FIVE

Sterilization and Prevention of Cross-infection

All dental treatments must be carried out under conditions which will reduce the dangers of cross-infection by the transmission of pathogenic micro-organisms both to and from the patient. Such contamination may occur via the surroundings, instruments, materials or the dental team themselves. *The DSA must remain alert to this ever-present hazard at all times, for everyone's health and safety in the dental surgery depend upon her constant and meticulous care in these matters.*

STERILIZATION

Sterilization is a most important factor in the prevention of cross-infection. Sterile means completely free from all forms of life. Sterilization is the production of sterility by the complete removal or destruction of living micro-organisms and their spores from instruments and other material and may be achieved by heat, chemical or irradiation methods.

Presterilization cleaning
The DSA must wear thick rubber gloves during this preliminary process to protect herself from accidental infection or scratches. The contaminated instruments should be soaked in a disinfectant solution before cleaning. They are then scrubbed with a detergent and water, and rinsed clean. This must be done thoroughly for any debris retained, such as dried blood, may act as a barrier to the sterilisation process.

Alternatively the dirty instruments may be placed immediately into a bath of disinfectant and detergent solution in an ultrasonic cleaner. They are then subjected to high-frequency vibration which breaks up and shakes off even minute particles, very thoroughly, in a few minutes. The detergent must be rinsed off before sterilization.

Sterilization by moist heat
Boiling water. When the instruments and utensils are boiled in water (100°C) for 15 minutes most pathogenic organisms are killed, but this method cannot

destroy some highly resistant spores and certain viruses. Thus boiling water will disinfect but not sterilize.

Autoclave. This is the most reliable method of sterilizing instruments, utensils and other equipment in the dental surgery. Water boils at 100°C at normal atmospheric pressure. If the water is heated in a closed container, such as an autoclave, the steam pressure and the temperature continue to rise as the system is heated until at a pressure of 2.2 bar (32 lbs per square inch) the temperature reaches 134°C. No living thing can survive after three minutes' exposure to steam at this temperature.

Steam under pressure can penetrate porous substances, but not airtight containers. The items to be sterilized are placed in perforated containers, loosely wrapped in special paper or put into special bags or packets. Steam corrosion of certain instruments after autoclaving can be prevented by wrapping them in paper impregnated with vapour-phase inhibitor or by treating metal instruments with special solutions, such as 1 per cent sodium nitrate. Wrappings and containers are sealed with heat-sensitive adhesive tape which changes colour when heated, thus distinguishing between treated and untreated packages (Bowie Dick Autoclave Tape).

The small autoclave works by electricity. The apparatus has to be 'topped up' with distilled water to the required level each morning. Before opening the door of the autoclave check that the pressure gauge registers zero. The door is then opened and the prepared packages and containers are loaded into the autoclave, taking care to allow sufficient space for steam to circulate between them (Fig. 5/1). The door is closed firmly, the locking mechanism engaged and the starting button or switch operated to set the automatic cycle in motion. The pressure will rise gradually, slowly if this is the first load of the day, but more rapidly when the apparatus has been preheated by previous operating cycles. The pressure should reach 2.2 bar at which time the thermometer should register 134°C and the timer should enable this condition to be maintained for well over the required three minutes. Finally the cycle is completed by the automatic release of the steam pressure, with the condensation of the steam back into water and a reduction of pressure. The door may then be opened safely and the still hot containers and packets removed with a heat resistant glove or special forceps. The open steam-circulation ports on autoclave containers should be closed to prevent contamination from the air. Large hospital and commercial autoclaves of the *downward displacement* or *high vacuum* types use chambers from which air can be exhausted (heated by dry steam from an external source). The precise working of different makes of autoclave can vary. A 'drying cycle' in the programme is valuable because it ensures that the sterile packages contain no moisture thus preserving sterility for a longer period.

The efficiency of the autoclave process can be checked by including with

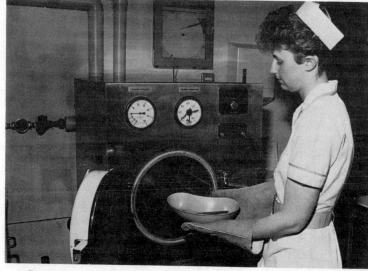

Fig. 5/1 Instruments being placed into a small steam autoclave prior to the
sterilization cycle

the load an indicator or 'teller' which shows a change when the required
temperature is reached, for example, Browne's indicator strips, or by
temperature monitors with a chart recorder.

Items that have been sterilized in this way may be stored in dry, dust-free
conditions in the dental surgery and the containers or packets opened as
required at a later date. Items wrapped in paper should be used within 3
months or else resterilized.

Sterilization by dry heat

Hot-air oven. Cleaned, heat-resistant equipment can be sterilized by subject-
ing it to hot air at a temperature of 160°C for 1 hour. Electrically heated hot-
air oven sterilizers have a thermometer, a thermostat and a timing switch so
that they can be set to operate under the required conditions.

Instruments are generally put into tape-sealed metal containers before
being placed in the oven. The load must be loosely packed to allow
circulation of air. Hot air is very useful for sterilizing sharp instruments and
root canal therapy boxes, though in the latter, paper points and cottonwool
may be discoloured by the heat. The load should be allowed to cool before it
is removed from the oven to avoid contaminated air being drawn into
contracting packages.

Molten metal, etc. Electrically heated containers are available which hold and heat up small quantities of molten metal, salt or glass beads to over 200°C. During root canal therapy small instruments and paper points held in tweezers may be dipped repeatedly into the heated material for 5 to 15 seconds to decontaminate their surfaces during treatment and thus help to disinfect the root canal. They have very limited application and are a source of danger if overturned.

Direct heat. Metal can be sterilized by heating it in a flame until it is red hot. This method is used in bacteriological investigations where a platinum wire loop is used to transfer infected material, such as pus, from one place to another. Such a wire loop is sterilized by holding it in a gas flame. Dental instruments would be ruined if heated in this way.

Sterilization by chemicals
Most germicidal chemicals are unsuitable for the purpose of sterilization. They have limited application and many spores and viruses are highly resistant to them for long periods.

Solutions. Certain items that would be damaged by heat can still be sterilized by immersing them in covered containers of cold sterilizing solutions such as 2 per cent activated gluteraldehyde. It is most important to follow the manufacturer's instructions precisely with regard to making up the solution, how often it must be changed, and the time required to achieve sterility. Items must be clean and dry before being put into the solution. Disinfection time is usually about 10 minutes, but sterilization will take several hours. Gluteraldehyde solutions give off irritant fumes which will affect the eyes and nose. The solution must be completely rinsed off instruments with sterile water before they are used, to avoid tissue irritation.

Gases. Certain equipment may be sterilized by exposing it to gases or vapours in a closed container. This method can be used in industry but is unsuitable for dental practice. The gases are:

1. Formaldehyde vapour, which has a poor capacity for penetration and a very slow sterilizing action.
2. Ethylene oxide gas, which is expensive, has a limited application and is highly explosive.

Sterilization by irradiation
Ionizing gamma radiation. This physical method is commonly used in industry to sterilize a wide range of disposable materials and equipment that is

obtainable in sealed packages and containers. A large, elaborate sterilizing plant is required with adequate safety precautions. The gamma radiation is obtained from radioactive sources such as cobalt 60. The rays can penetrate most materials and kill all organisms and spores very quickly. Disposable gloves, plastic surgical equipment, syringes, needles, suture materials, dressings, plasma, drugs destroyed by heat and so on may all be sterilized in this way.

Some particular problems of sterilization

Handpieces. In general, all handpieces can be sterilized in the autoclave (134°C) provided that the following special precautions are taken. They must first be thoroughly cleaned in the manner recommended by the manufacturer. It has been shown that lubricating oil remaining within the handpiece shields protects the spores of many organisms from the pressurized steam. This problem is overcome when the instrument has been treated by spraying a special penetrating additive into the retained oil which then vaporizes in the autoclave and destroys the organisms. Handpieces so treated are inserted into sealed containers or sachets before being placed in the autoclave so that they can be stored in a sterile condition until required. Handpieces can also be sterilized in a hot oven but the DSA should always check the manufacturer's instructions.

Air turbines. These can be sterilized in the autoclave after first removing the plastic bur chuck, and preferably after the above mentioned penetrating additive treatment. They must *not* be placed in the hot air oven because they will be damaged by the high temperature.

Glassware. This must be thoroughly cleaned with a detergent, rinsed and sterilized in the autoclave.

Glass clinical thermometers. These cannot be heated, but should be rinsed thoroughly in cold water and placed in a disinfectant solution. This solution should be changed frequently to ensure its effectiveness, and always rinsed off before the thermometer is used again. Alternatively, they may be disinfected in 70 per cent alcohol and stored dry.

Plastics. Equipment made of polyvinyl chloride (PVC), polytetrafluorethylene (PTFE) and polyethylene can be sterilized by autoclaving. New equipment should be boiled first in several changes of distilled water to remove any water-soluble traces in the plastic.

Polystyrene will melt at autoclave temperatures and can only be effectively sterilized with gamma rays or ethylene oxide gas. Acrylic (Perspex) is damaged by heat and gamma rays. Most chemical disinfectant solutions are absorbed by, or damage, heat-moulded plastics in the long run.

Rubber. Such equipment may be sterilized by autoclaving. New natural or silicone rubber apparatus should be boiled first in several changes of distilled water, as with plastics.

Central sterile supply department (CSSD)
Large hospitals use the CSSD system in which all used equipment is returned to one department for disposal or to be cleaned and sterilized before reissue. By concentrating all this work in one place the risk of cross-infection is reduced. The system requires duplication of many instruments and is thus too expensive for routine dental practice.

DENTAL TREATMENT AND ASEPSIS

In general, dental treatment may be divided into three main categories.

Surgical operations
In these the outer defensive tissues of the body are penetrated and the resultant wound is open to infection, for example, dental extraction, injection, root canal therapy. Any procedure that involves entry into the blood-carrying and serum-carrying tissues falls into the category. During all surgical procedures a strictly *aseptic technique* is essential and only sterile equipment may come into contact with the wound and its surrounding parts.

Asepsis is achieved when all living disease-causing micro-organisms have been killed or removed from the equipment in use and the immediate environment of the patient.

Non-surgical or routine treatment
The procedures in these cases do not penetrate the soft tissues, for example, impressions, simple conservation treatment, topical applications. During non-surgical treatment the normal routines of cleanliness and general hygiene must be observed to prevent cross-infection (to other patients and members of the dental team), but the strict aseptic techniques are not required.

Treatment of infections and high-risk patients
Special precautions are necessary when undertaking any kind of dental treatment for patients who are suffering from or are carriers of highly contagious diseases.

ASEPTIC TECHNIQUES

Environment
Air. Everything must be done to reduce airborne contamination. The surgery should be as dust-free as possible. The ventilation and heating should be planned to help in this respect. Ideally, surgery should be carried out in a special room set aside for that purpose and casual visitors forbidden, to prevent additional dust and organisms being brought in on their clothes, shoes, hair, skin and from the upper respiratory tract, etc. In an operating theatre the staff don special theatre boots and clean linen theatre clothes before entering the surgical areas.

Furniture and equipment. The walls and ceiling should be cleaned frequently and the floor washed daily. All dust-collecting surfaces should be washed frequently, ideally every day. The handbasin, taps and drains should be treated with disinfectant daily. General cleaning should be completed at least an hour before surgery to allow any remaining dust to settle. All metal and glass surfaces of dental equipment must be wiped over with a disinfecting solution between patients.

The dental team: theatre dress
Under ideal surgical conditions, in an operating theatre, both the dental surgeon and his assistant should change into theatre clothes, wear a mask and cap, special clean theatre boots or overshoes, waterproof apron, 'scrub up' their hands and don a sterile gown and rubber gloves before the operation begins. The extent to which this extreme standard of theatre dress is observed in the dental surgery will depend upon the decision of the individual dental surgeon and the type of operation being undertaken. Its absence must not be taken as a signal to relax the other rigid standards that are required to maintain the aseptic technique vital to safe surgery.

Mask. This may be of disposable paper or synthetic fibre. Masks are worn by the operating team to reduce the danger of infection from their mouths and upper respiratory tracts contaminating the wound. They are not perfect guards, for some micro-organisms can still pass through them. The operator and assistants should cover all cuts and abrasions on their own faces with waterproof dressings. The mask should be put into position before scrubbing the hands and not touched again until the operation is completed.

Cap. This must be worn so as to cover the hair completely and prevent organisms falling on to the wound from that source. The cap also should be put on before the hands are scrubbed. Caps are usually disposable.

Apron. In the theatre it is best to wear a disposable, waterproof apron, otherwise if the sterile gown is subsequently wetted with water or blood, this will soak through and the gown will become contaminated by the non-sterile clothing underneath.

Gown. The sterile operating gown is opened up carefully at arms' length taking care not to touch or contaminate the outside surfaces. The arms are slipped up into the sleeves and an assistant ties the neck tapes. The waist tapes should be held out sideways by their extreme ends so that an assistant can take them easily and tie them behind the waist.

Hands. The skin of the hands harbours many pathogenic micro-organisms and it cannot be sterilized. However well the surface of the skin is cleaned, perspiration brings hordes of new organisms to the surface from the depths of the sweat glands.

The hands should be well cared for at all times, with short nails and a healthy, unbroken skin. Any cuts or abrasions of the hands should be covered with waterproof adhesive plaster. 'Scrubbing-up' before an operation entails scrubbing the fingernails with a sterile brush for 1 minute and then washing the hands and forearms for 3 minutes using an antiseptic skin cleanser and a constant stream of warm water. Using such a cleanser, such as Hibitane, means that after the initial scrub for the first case on an operating list, the hands may be adequately cleaned by just washing them with cleanser and water for subsequent cases.

The hands are rinsed free of cleanser, keeping them raised above elbow level, and the taps turned off with the elbow, for now that the hands are clean they must not be contaminated by water from higher up the arms or contact with non-sterile surfaces. The hands, and then the arms, are dried carefully with a sterile towel.

Gloves. Rubber gloves, of various sizes, are provided in sterile wallets together with a packet of glove powder. The wallet is opened carefully, the powder packet extracted and its talc-like contents dusted over the hands and between the fingers. A small amount of powder may also be dusted into the interior of the gloves. One glove is removed from the wallet, holding it by its folded-back cuff, so that only the *inside* of the glove is touched by the skin, and slipped on to the hand. The second glove is now removed by slipping the fingers of the gloved hand underneath the folded-back cuff so that only the *outside* of the second glove is touched by the first. The second hand is inserted into the glove. Finally the cuffs of the gloves are unfolded back to cover and grip the gown sleeves, making sure that the gloved fingers only come into contact with the *outside* of the sterile gloves and are not contaminated from the skin surfaces. In an alternative 'closed' method of donning rubber gloves the gown sleeves are first pulled down to cover the scrubbed hands before the gloves are touched at all.

Having reached this stage the members of the operating team must not touch a non-sterile surface or object (apart from the operation site) for if they do they must retire from the scene of the operation and carry out the 'scrubbing-up' process again.

Instruments and materials

Sterile instruments and materials must be set out by the 'no touch' technique which can only be learnt by actual practice. Clean tables and trolleys may be set out by first covering them with a sterile waterproof sheet then a sterile towel and then placing sterile instruments, dressings and containers, such as gallipots and kidney dishes, on the towel as required. Sealed paper packages of instruments may be torn open at one end and their contents slid out, untouched, on to the sterile towel or into a sterile dish. A laid-up trolley may be further protected until it is required by covering it with another sterile towel.

The patient

In the operating theatre the patient is draped with sterile waterproof sheeting covered with sterile towels held in place with sterile towel clips so that only the operation site, the mouth, is left exposed. The skin around the mouth and the oral mucosa may be cleaned with non-irritant antiseptic solutions.

In the dental surgery the patient's outdoor clothing and hair may be covered in a similar way. In the conscious patient saliva flowing near the operation site may be kept clear with adequate suction through a sterile sucker tip (Fig. 5/2). Wounds must *never* be irrigated with water from the dental unit sprays but only with sterile water or saline delivered by sterilized syringe or drip system.

ROUTINE DENTAL TREATMENT

Traditionally most attention has been focused on the methods of protecting the patient undergoing surgical treatment in order to avoid wound infections, etc., and in taking special precautions to protect the clinical staff in cases of known transmissible disease. Recently, however, attention has been increasingly directed towards the hazards of transmitting certain diseases, particularly hepatitis B and AIDS (see Chapter 18) during routine dental treatment. For example, in the former case, patients who suffer the disease both clinically or subclinically and recover, may remain in a 'carrier' state for the rest of their lives. Such carriers, although apparently quite healthy in

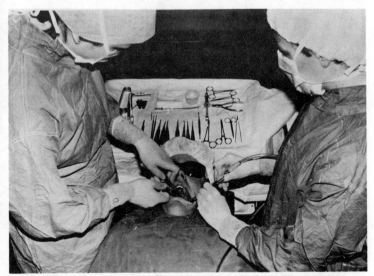

Fig. 5/2 An oral surgery procedure under strictly aseptic conditions. The DSA is maintaining good visibility using a narrow suction tip to draw off blood and irrigating saline, and by retracting tissues as directed by the operator

themselves are a constant source of danger to others in that they may transmit the disease to them. This can be done via minute quantities of blood, saliva, and other body fluids. Thus every dental surgeon and his clinical team has been advised to treat all patients as if they were carriers in order to protect themselves and all other patients and visitors to the practice. The techniques that must be employed, even for the most routine dental care, are quite demanding, but once learnt they soon become a routine part of safe everyday practice.

Sequence for good dental practice
It is recommended that the following sequences of good dental practice are carried out for all patients. Where extra procedures are required for the treatment of known high-risk cases these are indicated with an asterisk (*).

1. All members of the clinical dental team should be vaccinated against hepatitis B (see Chapter 18).
2. Change out of clothes and shoes worn outside the surgery before a clinical session (thus infection will not be carried home). Do not wear rings, jewellery or a wrist-watch in the surgery as they prevent thorough

cleaning of the hands and are a source of cross-infection. Wear a clean coat every day. *Change the coat or gown after treating a contagious patient.

3. Ensure that the sterilizing system is working properly and is being used correctly, for example, presterilization cleaning.

   Arrange to use disposable items as much as possible, such as towels, plastic mouthwash cups, saliva ejectors, needles, cartridges, scalpels, polishing brushes, etc. *Never re-use disposable items*.

4. A thorough medical history must be taken from every patient and updated on subsequent visits.

5. *All patients who may constitute a risk of infection, such as known carriers of contagious disease, should be treated at the *end* of the session to allow adequate time for cleaning the surgery thoroughly afterwards. This cleaning can be made easier by prior planning and rehearsal, and by protecting working surfaces and switches with disposable clingfilm plastic sheet. Have a container of 1 per cent sodium hypochlorite solution (Milton or Domestos) and a disposable cloth ready to deal with infectious spillages.

   *For contagious patients both the surgeon and the DSA must wear a plastic apron, a theatre gown and cap, gloves, mask and eye protection. These, of course, must be changed after each case and spectacles cleaned appropriately.

6. Both operator and DSA should wear disposable rubber gloves for all patients. At present it is presumed that the gloves can be cleaned adequately between patients by washing them with soap, detergent or hand cleanser. However, new gloves for each patient should be considered. Cuts or breaks in the skin should be covered with waterproof adhesive plaster before putting the gloves on. Never touch your face or hair during treatment, because of the danger of crossinfection.

7. Protective glasses or other eye protection and a face mask should be worn whenever there is a risk of aerosol spray or splashes from air rotors or scaling instruments. *Such aerosol-producing apparatus should never be used if any member of the surgery staff is not immune to hepatitis.

8. Use efficient aspiration to remove the aerosols from air rotors and ultrasonic scalers. Ensure that the aspirator exhausts out of the surgery into the open. Keep the surgery well ventilated. *Keep aerosols to a minimum. *The three-in-one water and air syringe must not be used unless the tip can be removed for sterilization.

9. Impressions should be washed and treated with disinfectant solution (depending upon the type of impression material) before sending them to the laboratory. *For infectious patients it is recommended that silicone materials are used so that they can then be soaked in glutar-

aldehyde solution for several hours. This can be done in the surgery, or the impressions may be sealed in plastic bags and labelled 'biohazard' for appropriate transmission to the previously notified dental laboratory. *Disposable trays should be employed and if tried in the mouth must be either used or destroyed. Appliances, such as dentures, should also be disinfected before sending them to the dental laboratory.

10. Hands should always be washed again after removing gloves and gown. Any area of intact skin that might have been contaminated with blood should be washed thoroughly but nothing done to cause bleeding. It is not necessary to scrub the skin or use strong disinfectants or detergents.

11. Great care must be taken to avoid accidental 'needlestick' injuries. Any puncture wounds must be encouraged to bleed freely and then washed with hand cleanser and water. If a splash of blood or infected material enters the DSA's eye or mouth it must also be washed away thoroughly with copious water. Any accident of this sort must be reported to the dental surgeon and medical advice sought immediately. (Check with the local district medical officer (DMO) or dental officer (DDO) for recommended referral for advice in such cases.)

12. Disinfect all working surfaces and equipment controls after use by wiping them with alcohol, or, if there are blood splashes, with a 1 per cent solution of sodium hypochlorite, or in the case of metal, 2 per cent glutaraldlehyde solution. Wear thick gloves while clearing up like this at the end of the day or *after a high-risk case. Flush through the aspirator and saliva tubing with the recommended disinfectant for your equipment and leave it overnight.

13. Disposal of infected items: sharp instruments, such as needles, scalpels, etc., together with used local anaesthetic cartridges should be collected into a rigid 'sharps' container and sealed. Used dressings, cottonwool rolls, etc., go into strong or double plastic bags and sealed. Both are to be collected under local arrangements (check with the DDO or dental committee) or incinerated. *These items must never go into the dustbin for domestic refuse collection.*

14. Gowns can be laundered in a hot wash cycle at 90°C. *Contaminated gowns or clothes should be collected into a sealed plastic bag in the surgery immediately after the patient leaves and labelled for special attention. Disposable gowns are recommended when treating high-risk patients.

15. Keep the practice policy for the prevention of cross-infection up to date. Discuss it at regular intervals with all the members of the clinical team, and do not forget to include the others in the practice such as the cleaner who may have a vital part to play. Make sure that new members of staff joining the team are fully indoctrinated with the policy before they start work.

If these procedures are adopted for all patients, it is possible for clinically healthy carriers of hepatitis B and AIDS, even if the condition has not been diagnosed or revealed, to be treated safely in general practice. However, dental patients who are ill or jaundiced should be referred to a hospital dental department who have appropriate facilities.

CHAPTER SIX

Dental Records and Charting

THE DENTAL RECORD

Case history taking, clinical examination, diagnostic tests and treatment planning together form the foundation of all successful dental care. Accurate and up-to-date records of every stage of examination and treatment are essential to ensure continuity of treatment and to protect the dental surgeon in the unlikely event of legal proceedings by a dissatisfied patient. Most dental surgeons follow a methodical system such as:

1. Name
2. Age
3. Address and telephone number
4. Occupation
5. Name and address of general medical practitioner
6. PMH (previous medical history)
7. PDH (previous dental history)
8. C/O (patient complains of . . .)
9. O/E (on examination)
      extraoral
      intraoral (includes making a chart of the teeth)
10. Provisional diagnosis
      Special tests (to investigate further)
11. Firm diagnosis
12. Treatment plan (immediate and long-term)

The DSA must be prepared to write down all these details as they are dictated to her by the dental surgeon, unless he prefers to make this record himself.

The dental chart

This is the most important record of the patient's dental condition. Usually the dental surgeon calls out the teeth, stating the cavities, fillings and so on as he discovers them during his intraoral examination and the DSA makes an accurate representation of the presence and condition of the teeth by filling in symbols and outlines on a standard chart of the mouth (Figs 6/1 and 6/2).

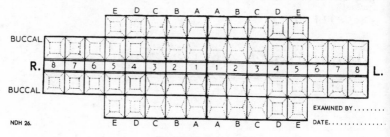

Fig. 6/1 Teeth chart

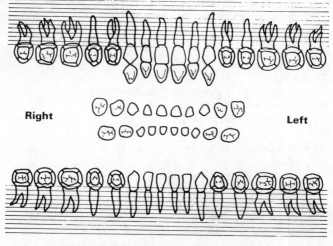

Fig. 6/2 Anatomical chart for periodontal records

The 32 permanent teeth and the 20 primary teeth can be described in words or numerical symbols.

The quadrant system
In this commonly used system, the mouth is divided into four segments and the teeth are designated as follows:

Permanent teeth

```
                        UPPER

              87654321 │ 12345678
    RIGHT ─────────────┼─────────────── LEFT
              87654321 │ 12345678

                        LOWER
```

Primary teeth

```
                        UPPER

               EDCBA │ ABCDE
    RIGHT ────────────┼──────────── LEFT
               EDCBA │ ABCDE

                        LOWER
```

It should be noted that 'right' and 'left' are the *patient's* right and left.

In this way individual teeth can be described as in the following examples:

'Upper right five' = $\underline{5}\rfloor$ = upper right second premolar

'Lower left one' = $\lceil\overline{1}$ = lower left central incisor

'Upper left C' = $\lfloor\underline{C}$ = upper left primary canine

The two-digit system

This international system for designating teeth is used by some dental surgeons, mostly outside Great Britain, because it simplifies the handling and communication of dental data, for example, in computer programming. The quadrants are allocated digits 1 to 4 for permanent teeth in a clockwise sequence on the chart starting at the right upper side:

Permanent teeth

			Upper right								Upper left				
18	17	16	15	14	13	12	11	21	22	23	24	25	26	27	28
48	47	46	45	44	43	42	41	31	32	33	34	35	36	37	38
			Lower right								Lower left				

Primary teeth

	Upper right						Upper left			
55	54	53	5²	51		61	62	63	64	65
85	84	83	82	81		71	7²	73	74	75
	Lower right						Lower left			

Examples:

'One-two'	$= 12 =$	upper right second incisor
'Three-eight'	$= 38 =$	lower left third molar
'Five-four'	$= 54 =$	upper right first primary molar

The surfaces of the teeth. These are described by their anatomical names. Sometimes the words describing the surfaces involved in a cavity are abbreviated to their initial letters: for example, mesio-occluso-distal, disto-occlusal or occluso-buccal become MOD, DO or OB.

The standard charts are usually diagrammatic (see Fig. 6/1) but occasionally the crowns of the teeth are anatomically represented. Other charts are available for specialized purposes. In periodontal treatment a representation of the roots of the teeth will be necessary to record the depths of any pockets around the teeth (see Fig. 6/2). In cases of fracture of the jaws a representation of the whole skull will enable the surgeon to keep an accurate record of gross bony injuries.

Common charting symbols

The following are used:

Tooth present and sound	.
Tooth partially erupted	pe
Tooth unerupted	u
Tooth missing	—
Tooth to be extracted	/
Tooth recently extracted	×
Root present	+
Cavity	○
Filling	●
Unsound filling present to be restored	◉
Tooth root filled	RF
Tooth non-vital	NV
Artificial tooth present	A
Crown present	C
Indicating the direction and extent of movement of teeth	→

Bridge retainer present	BR
Bridge pontic present	BP
Gold inlay	GI

Primary teeth are indicated in the top right-hand corner of the appropriate square as ABCDE in diagrammatic charts without special provision for them.

Treatment records

A brief record of the treatment carried out must be made immediately after the patient leaves the surgery while it is still fresh in the mind. This should indicate the exact region, tooth or tooth surface involved, what was done, and what materials or drugs were used. Any untoward occurrences during treatment must be recorded in full detail.

Abbreviations. These are often used in practice, for example, '$\overline{6|}$ -MO ACR ID 2 % Xyl' means 'a Class II, mesio-occlusal cavity was prepared in the lower right first permanent molar under inferior dental block anaesthesia obtained with 2 per cent xylocaine solution. The cavity was lined with cement and restored with amalgam.'

The following list gives other examples of abbreviations commonly used but they are not themselves standard and may vary from practice to practice. The DSA must use and interpret them *very carefully* to avoid mistakes.

A	Amalgam
Ac	Acrylic
Ag	Silver
ANK	Appointment not kept
Au	Gold
C	Cement
DNA	Did not attend
F/- or FU	Complete upper denture
-/F or FL	Complete lower denture
F/F	Complete dentures
GA	General anaesthetic
GDP	General dental practitioner
GMP	General medical practitioner
GP	Gutta percha
HSWMW	Hot salt water mouthwash
ID	Inferior dental block injection
Imps	Impressions
Inf	Infiltration injection
LA	Local anaesthetic
P/- or PU	Partial upper denture

-/P or PL	Partial lower denture
QS	Quick set
R	Restoration
RCT	Root canal therapy
SM	Study models
TCA	To come again
TP	Treatment plan
TTP	Tender to percussion
X	Extraction
ZnO	Zinc oxide (dressing)
#	Fracture (this sign also means 'number', e.g. #4)
⑥	Abscess (number denotes the tooth involved)

Other records

Various special diagnostic tests may be undertaken and the results must be carefully recorded and filed or stored as they become available.

Radiographs. Radiographs must always be labelled with the patient's name and the date upon which they were taken before they are filed. This also applies to photographic records.

Bulky records. Study models, specifically indicated working models, discarded dentures, etc., should be stored in labelled boxes to protect them from dust or breakage.

Laboratory tests. The results of laboratory investigation (biopsies, blood tests, bacteriological smears) should always be brought to the dental surgeon's immediate attention before they are filed away with the patient's records.

CHAPTER SEVEN

Dental Radiography

X-RAYS

X-rays are a radiation comparable to light and radio waves but differing from them in wavelength. They travel in a straight line from their source and can penetrate materials that are opaque to light, being deflected or absorbed by heavy atoms such as those found in metal and yet able to penetrate lighter atoms.

X-ray apparatus

X-rays are generated when a stream of electrons is stopped by impact with a solid. Inside a glass vacuum tube a heated wire filament (the cathode) generates a cloud of electrons which are accelerated by a high voltage electrical potential towards a shaped mass of metal (the anode) and focused upon its surface. The energy of their impact generates x-rays which are emitted in all directions. Heat is also produced at the anode and so exposures are kept very short in duration and the vacuum tube is surrounded by a cooling jacket containing oil.

The tube is housed in a heavy metal screening cover which has a small window through which the working beam of x-rays is allowed to escape. The diameter of this beam can be limited and stopped down by a lead diaphragm and the central ray of the beam is arranged to pass through the point of a plastic centring cone on the x-ray machine's working head. The working head, which contains and covers the tube and its housing, is supported in a carefully counterbalanced positioning device that allows great flexibility of movement and angulation.

The apparatus has two warning lights: one to show that the machine is connected to the electrical mains and is 'live'; the second is a prominent and clearly visible indication of when x-rays are being generated. The x-ray set must be properly maintained to ensure that it does not continue to produce x-rays after the preset exposure has ended. The machine should always be switched off and 'dead' when not in use.

Dangers of exposure to x-rays

People working with x-rays are recommended to wear an exposure mon-itoring film badge to check that radiological safety standards are being maintained. Advice about such badges can be obtained from the local department of medical physics.

Prolonged exposure to x-rays is very dangerous and the operator and others must make sure that they protect themselves by avoiding the direct beam and standing at least 1.8 m (6 feet) away from the tube during exposures. No-one other than the patient and the operator should remain in an x-ray room during the exposure unless this is essential, for example the mother to reassure a child. The x-ray beam should not be directed through thin walls into other areas or premises. Patients must not be exposed to x-rays beyond one full mouth-examination (10 to 14 intraoral films) a year, unless diagnostically necessary.

The x-ray beam should not be angled through the patient's trunk and must be directed away from the gonads. A pregnant woman patient should not be exposed *at all* to x-rays in the dental surgery if it can be avoided because of the danger to the developing cells of the unborn child. When an x-ray is essential in such a case, the mother and child must be protected with a special lead-rubber protective apron.

In no circumstances must the operator touch the cone or the tube housing, or hold a film in position in a patient's mouth during an exposure because the cumulative effects of such x-ray exposures can lead to radiation burns, skin ulceration, necrosis (death) of bone and loss of fingers.

In Great Britain the dental surgeon is accepted as a recognized radiation worker allowed to use x-rays in the dental surgery. The DSA may assist while radiographs are being taken, but is *not allowed* to use x-rays herself unless adequately trained and supervised.

(*Note:* Exposure to the x-ray beam can 'de-program' and spoil certain digital watches.)

Films

Ordinary photographic emulsion is sensitive to both light and x-rays. If a film, protected from light and moisture, is placed in the mouth on one side of the teeth and a beam of x-rays directed towards it from the other side, it passes through the teeth, bone and other tissues and throws a varying shadow on the film. The exposed film can then be developed in the dark room by ordinary photographic methods and will disclose details of the structures in and around the teeth that could not otherwise be examined.

Films may be *intraoral* (for example, periapical, occlusal, bite-wing) or *extraoral* (for example, lateral oblique, lateral skull, orthopantomogram (OPT)).

Intraoral films. The dental film packet for intraoral use is supplied made up as follows (see also Fig. 7/4):

1. A thin piece of tough transparent plastic film coated on both sides with a fine-grain photographic emulsion sandwiched between two thin sheets of black paper. (Some packets contain two pieces of film and the duplicate obtained is used for record purposes.)
2. This film is backed by a sheet of thin lead foil to prevent the x-rays from passing further and perhaps being reflected back from nearby structures and spoiling the film.
3. The outer envelope is made of lightproof paper and is labelled to indicate the side which should face away from the x-ray tube. This envelope is made up so that it can be opened easily in the dark room. (Some new films are contained in a simple plastic envelope only.)
4. In one corner of the film and repeated on the outer packet, there is a raised dot or pimple on the side that has to be towards the tube during exposure. This is of help in orientating the processed film correctly for viewing.

Extraoral films. Large extraoral films are usually exposed in lightproof, rigid metal cases called *cassettes.* When using extraoral film, the x-rays have to pass through much denser areas of bone in the skull and, in order to increase their effect on the film without increasing the exposure time considerably, *intensifying screens* are fixed inside the cassette. These screens contain certain chemicals that glow and fluoresce when struck by x-rays right inside the light-proof cassette and this light further affects the film.

Extraoral films must be orientated with a small lead letter 'L' or 'R' attached to the outside of the cassette before the exposure to indicate left or right. This letter will then be reproduced on the processed film.

All unexposed or undeveloped film must be protected from accidental x-ray radiation that will spoil it.

Making an exposure
1. The x-ray apparatus is switched on. Most machines are provided with a mains supply regulator so that the voltage may be adjusted to the recommended level before use.
2. The patient's head is positioned, resting it against a rigid support, such as the head rest of the dental chair.
3. The tube is placed in approximate position.
4. The film is placed in position.
5. The tube is adjusted to its accurate position.
6. The hand-timer, attached to the apparatus by a long cable, is set for the appropriate exposure time.
7. The operator and others retire to an appropriate distance behind the tube.

8. A visual check is made that nothing has moved, and the patient is warned to remain still.
9. The exposure release button is pressed firmly, noting that the exposure warning light on the apparatus comes on or, where provided, the milliammeter registers, while the exposure is made.
10. The intraoral film is removed from the mouth and wiped dry as soon as possible to prevent saliva soaking through the paper envelope and affecting the film.

Exposure time will vary with the machine, the speed of the film that is used and the tissue penetration required. For example, with the average dental apparatus with an x-ray output at 10mA and 60kV, using a 22.5 cm (9 inch) focus-to-film distance and a fast film, intraoral periapical films can be taken using exposures as short as 0.25 to 0.50 seconds.

Film positioning:
Periapical films
1. The occlusal plane of the jaw to be radiographed should be horizontal.
2. The film packet is supported on the palatal or lingual side of the tooth with a special holder or forceps, so that the margin of the film just projects beyond the occlusal edge of the tooth and its sensitive side is towards the tube. The orientation pimple on the film packet should be kept towards the occlusal margin.
3. The tooth and the film are not parallel and to reduce distortion the central ray from the tube is directed at right angles to the plane, bisecting the angle between the axis of the tooth and the film (Fig. 7/1). The

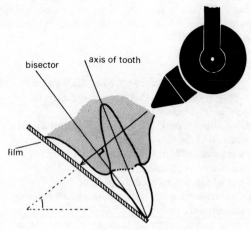

Fig. 7/1 Film and tube positioned for periapical radiography

approximate vertical angle between the horizontal occlusal plane and the central ray for the various upper and lower teeth is shown in the chart below.

Between 10 and 14 films are required to give full-mouth periapical radiographs depending upon the system used to position the films.

Upper teeth	Vertical angle of x-ray tube	Lower teeth	Vertical angle of x-ray tube
1̄	+55°	1̄	−20°
2̄3̄	+50°	2̄3̄	−20°
4̄5̄6̄	+30°	4̄5̄6̄	−10°
7̄8̄	+20°	7̄8̄	− 5°

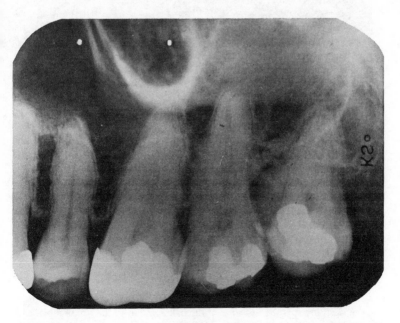

Fig. 7/2 Periapical radiography 5 6 7 8

Bite-wing films. A bite-wing film is obtained using a standard intraoral film packet which has a paper flange or special holder attached to it along the occlusal plane. This holder is gripped between the teeth thus supporting the film firmly against the lingual and palatal surfaces of the upper and lower teeth at the same time. The tube is positioned with a 0° vertical angle from the occlusal plane. Only the crowns of the teeth will be shown on this film (Fig. 7/3).

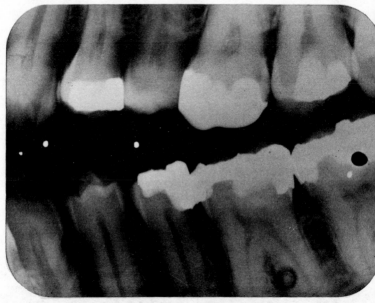

Fig. 7/3 Bite-wing radiograph (left side)

Occlusal films. These are taken with larger intraoral film packets held lightly between the occlusal surfaces of the upper and lower teeth with the sensitive side of the packet towards the tube.

The standard upper occlusal film. The central ray is directed from the bridge of the nose towards the mid-line of the palate at an angle of 60° to the occlusal plane.

The true upper occlusal film. The central ray is directed through the vertex of the skull towards the mid-line of the palate at 90° to the occlusal plane. A longer exposure time is required.

The lower occlusal film. The patient's head is extended and the tube is aimed upwards from below the chin at 90° to the occlusal plane.

Extraoral films. These require larger films used in a cassette. The lateral oblique film is commonly taken to examine the molar region and ramus of the mandible. The cassette is supported against the angle of the mandible and cheek with the patient's head tilted as well as turned towards that side. The central ray can now be directed below the opposite angle of the mandible towards the molar region of the side under examination.

Other extraoral films occasionally required include full lateral and posteroanterior skull films, films to show the maxillary antra (singular: antrum) and views of the temporomandibular joint.

Film processing
See Fig. 7/4.

The exposed dental film or *radiograph* is processed in the same way as ordinary photographic film, usually in the dark room although daylight tanks or processors may be used in special circumstances.

Exposed films are *developed* with chemical solutions that carry on the work begun by the action of light or x-rays. The silver salts in the photographic emulsion that have been affected by the exposure are reduced to fine grains of metallic silver and then the film is *fixed* by further chemical action to remove the non-affected, unexposed silver salts in the other areas of the film.

Dark room procedures
The dark room excludes all normal daylight or artificial light that would affect the light-sensitive photographic emulsion. The only permissible light is from a special dim safelight fitted with an amber filter. Once one's eyes have become accustomed to this low glow the light is adequate for film processing procedures.

The standard solutions in the processing tanks must be well mixed and replaced regularly according to the manufacturer's instructions. The temperature of the solutions is important and should be checked with a thermometer and when necessary a special electric tank heater can be used.

When the dark room has been prepared the films are processed in the following way.

1. Lock the dark room door.
2. Switch off the ordinary light and put on the safelight.
3. Make sure that your hands are dry and clean.
4. Open the film containers one by one and clip the films in sequence on to the photographic hanger. Take care to hold the films by their edges only

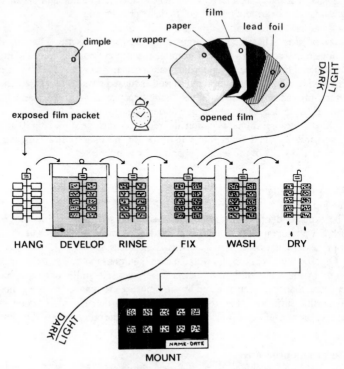

Fig. 7/4 Stages in processing intraoral dental films

to avoid touching the emulsion. Up to 14 films may be placed on one hanger.

5. Label the hanger with the patient's name.
6. Put the discarded packet papers and lead foil into the appropriate waste receivers.
7. Put the films into the developer tank and agitate the hanger a little to prevent bubbles of air from remaining on the film surfaces and impeding the chemical action.
8. Put the lightproof lid on top of the developing tank.
9. Set the timing clock to indicate the developing time. This will be about 4 minutes at 20°C but depends upon the film speed, so check carefully.
10. When the developing time has elapsed lift the films from the developing tank and wash them in running water in the rinsing tank for 10 seconds to stop the chemical action.

11. Place the washed films into the fixing tank, again agitating them to remove air bubbles.
12. Reset the timing clock to indicate the fixing time. This varies from 5 to 10 minutes, depending upon the chemical used.
13. When the films are fixed they are no longer light-sensitive and the dim light can be exchanged for normal lighting.
14. After fixing, the films are washed well in running water to remove all traces of chemicals and then hung up to dry in a dust-free atmosphere.

Note: Automatic film processing machines are now available to develop dental x-ray films. They require careful maintenance to ensure that the rollers are washed and clean and that the solutions are replaced regularly.

Faults
The following are some faults commonly met with and their most likely causes:

Film too dark: overexposure or overdevelopment
Film too light: underexposure or underdevelopment
No image: x-ray machine not switched on or fixing tank was inadvertently used first
Partial image: film in contact with another in tank
Fogged film: old film stock or light leak in dark room
Stained film: inadequate fixing or washing
Double image: patient or tube moved during exposure
Curved dark lines: film damaged by bending it

Orientating and mounting films
Intraoral films are embossed in one corner with a raised pimple that is convex towards the tube (or the front of the film packet). By looking at the film as if from the outside of the patient's mouth, using the pimple as a guide, it is possible to orientate the film by the anatomy of the teeth depicted. Some dental surgeons store films in small envelopes while others prefer the films to be mounted on special sheets of transparent plastic or in cardboard mounts in their appropriate orientated positions for easy examination on the illuminated viewing box. Always write the patient's name on the envelope or mount *immediately*.

CHAPTER EIGHT

Basic Conservative Dentistry

Conservative dentistry is concerned with the operative techniques and materials used to restore carious, broken or worn natural teeth to normal function. More than half the time spent at the chairside in general practice is devoted to this type of treatment. This important and intricate work has to be carried out in the confined, dark, wet and sensitive environment of the mouth where each new restoration is immediately subjected to the destructive effects of masticatory pressures, moisture, temperature changes, various chemical activities and even the possibility of secondary carious attack. Instruments, materials and methods have been evolved to minimize or overcome these formidable difficulties.

THE OPERATING FIELD

The operating field has to be made as accessible and clearly visible as possible by positioning the patient's head properly, illuminating the mouth well, using a mouth mirror when necessary and by keeping the area dry. (Mouth mirrors may have plane or magnifying surfaces.)

Methods to keep teeth dry
A tooth can be kept dry by a variety of methods.

The saliva ejector (low volume suction). This has an appropriate tip attached; it will evacuate saliva from the mouth slowly, and works by water pressure.

The aspirator (high volume suction). This has a saliva ejector tip and a separate suction tip directed towards the tooth by the assistant. This will rapidly evacuate saliva, water and aerosol sprays from the mouth, and works by a vacuum generated by an electric pump.

Absorbent pads (for example, cotton wool rolls). These are placed in the buccal, labial or lingual sulcus to absorb saliva. These will work best when they are positioned near the appropriate salivary duct to absorb the saliva at its source.

The rubber dam. A thin sheet of rubber is perforated with a rubber dam punch (Fig. 8/1) and applied to the appropriate teeth so that they protrude through the prepared holes. The sheet is retained on the teeth by special spring clamps or ligatured in place with waxed thread around the necks of the teeth. The edges of the dam are controlled by fastening them to a frame holder. The isolated teeth are thus kept free of moisture and contamination from the rest of the mouth during treatment and this method is commonly used during root canal therapy. The dam also prevents the patient from accidentally swallowing or inhaling small instruments.

Air drying and wiping. The teeth may be dried by blowing warm air on them from an air syringe or by wiping them with a pledget of cottonwool held in tweezers.

Antisialogogues. On rare occasions the mouth and teeth can be made drier if before the operation the patient is given a drug to reduce salivary flow.

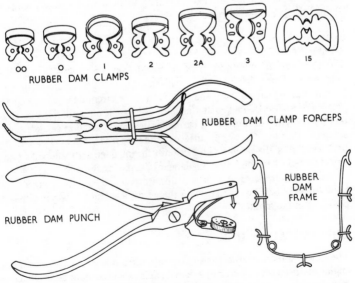

Fig. 8/1 Rubber dam instruments

HAND INSTRUMENTS

Dental probes
See Fig. 8/2.
These are sharp, pointed instruments that are made with a wide selection of curves and bends in their terminal shafts so that the tip may be more easily carried into remote places in the mouth. They are used in conservative dentistry primarily to explore tooth surfaces, to locate cavities and wide pits and fissures and to search the prepared cavity surfaces to ensure that all traces of softened carious tooth substance have been eliminated.

Chisels
See Fig. 8/3.
These are used to split off unsupported enamel along the cleavage planes parallel to the enamel's prisms and also to plane down and smooth the cavity margins. Each type of chisel is made so that its cutting edge can be easily applied to the particular surface of the cavity for which it is intended. A *straight* chisel is exactly comparable with a wood-worker's chisel, although it is many times smaller, with the shaft in a straight line with the handle. *Angled* or *bin-angled* (having two bends or angles in the shaft) chisels are either *hoe* chisels (with their edge at right angles to the main shaft as in a garden hoe) or *hatchet* chisels (with their cutting edge in line with the main shaft like an axe). *Gingival margin trimmers* are hatchet chisels adapted for use in planning the cervical margins of interproximal cavities.

Excavators
See Fig. 8/4.
Softened, carious dentine can be removed from cavities by using hand excavators. These have small, spoon-shaped, circular (discoid) or oval (cleoid) tips which are very sharp around their circumference. They are pressed into the carious material and used to lever and dig out large fragments. When the bulk of the caries has been removed they can be used to scrape and explore the firmer surface of the prepared tooth to eliminate any final fragments. They allow good visibility during deep excavation of a tooth and are used when there is some danger of exposing the pulp.

Many different sizes of excavator tips are available and there are several basic angles of terminal shaft to allow them to be used more easily in different positions in the mouth.

THE DENTAL ENGINE

The quickest method of preparing cavities in teeth is by the use of rotating engine instruments powered by a dental engine that is usually controlled by a foot switch.

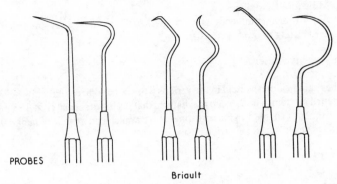

PROBES

Briault

Fig. 8/2 Dental probes

Electric engine
This is a variable-speed electric motor which drives the handpiece. Instrument speeds of from less than 500rpm up to 25 000rpm can be obtained and in some cases, specially geared engines connected to handpieces with high-speed bearings can be adjusted to develop 100 000rpm. It is now almost entirely superseded by the air-driven engines.

Air motor
This engine drive is directly adjacent to the handpiece and the motive power is produced by a slow air turbine fed by a simple tube conveying compressed air. This power system is very simple and the handpiece is relatively unrestricted in movement.

Air turbine
The motive power is again produced by compressed air passing through a turbine but now the turbine is a high-speed one and is actually in the head of the handpiece. Very high speeds of 250 000rpm to 300 000rpm can be obtained with this system and the handpiece bearings have to be lubricated constantly during use by a fine oil mist produced by dripping oil into the air-feed line.

Handpieces
See Fig. 8/5.
These are of various types and are used to hold the engine-driven instrument firmly and transmit the motive power of the engine to it. They may be:

1. Straight handpieces
2. Right-angled handpieces
3. Contra-angled handpieces

4. Miniature handpieces
5. Air turbine handpieces (always used with a water spray to prevent overheating of the tooth).

Engine instruments

See Fig. 8/6.

These are made to be held in the various types of handpieces either by being gripped in a chuck or by a clip mechanism that fits into a special groove in the instrument's shank. Engine instruments are available in a range of materials and shapes to suit their various uses.

Materials

1. Steel
2. Hardened tungsten carbide steel
3. A steel shaft with a working head covered in diamond particles
4. A steel shaft carrying a carborundum point or stone
5. A steel mandrel to which may be attached a wide variety of discs or wheels (such as carborundum, diamond, rubber, sandpaper)
6. A steel shaft carrying a bristle brush or rubber tip.

Shapes

1. Burs (Fig. 8/7): fissure (cross-cut fissure, tapered fissure), round (rose-head), inverted cone, wheel, end-cutting, finishing (which are smoother: round, pear, oval, flame-shaped).
2. Diamond instruments: bur shapes, fissure, round (rosehead), inverted cone, end-cutting both for conventional handpieces and air-rotors, wheels, discs, points.
3. Stones: green abrasive points, wheels and discs and white abrasive finishing points in many patterns.
4. Brushes and rubber polishing tips: cup and wheel shapes.

CAVITY CLASSIFICATION

Cavities in teeth are generally classified according to the site of commencement of the carious process, as first proposed by Dr G. V. Black.

Black's classification

Class I: Cavities originating in anatomical pits, fissures and structural defects

Class II: Cavities originating on the proximal surfaces of molars and premolars

Class III: Cavities originating on the proximal surfaces of the incisors and canines and not involving the incisal angle

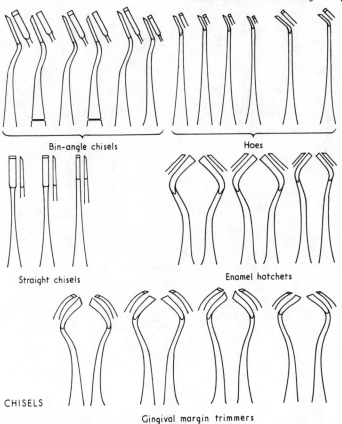

Bin-angle chisels

Hoes

Straight chisels

Enamel hatchets

CHISELS

Gingival margin trimmers

Fig. 8/3 Dental chisels

m.D. on to incisor edge

Class IV: Cavities originating on the proximal surfaces of incisors and canines and involving the incisal angle

Class V: Cavities originating on the gingival third of the labial, buccal, lingual or palatal surfaces of the teeth.

ingavie.

CAVITY PREPARATION

The last decade has seen a change in the philosophy of cavity preparation that had, for many years, closely adhered to the basic steps and designs set out by Black at the beginning of the century. Changes in the caries rate and diagnostic techniques plus improved preventive methods and new restora-

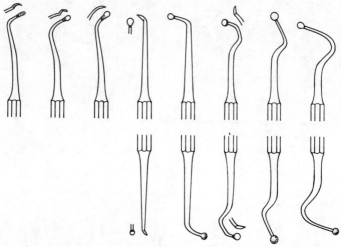

Fig. 8/4 Dental excavators

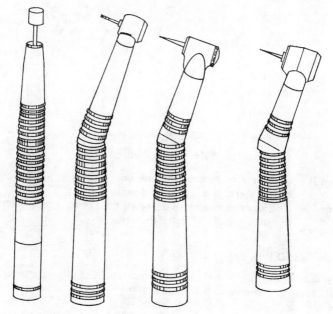

Fig. 8/5 Handpieces

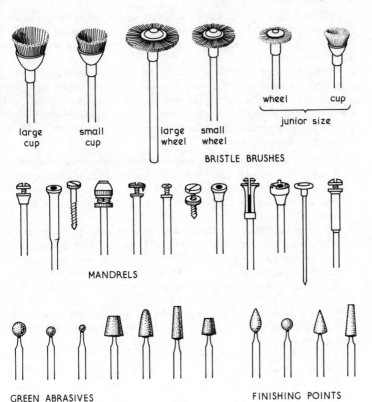

large cup small cup large wheel small wheel wheel cup

junior size

BRISTLE BRUSHES

MANDRELS

GREEN ABRASIVES FINISHING POINTS

Fig. 8/6 Engine instruments

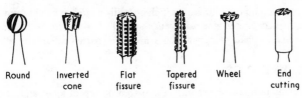

Round Inverted cone Flat fissure Tapered fissure Wheel End cutting

Fig. 8/7 Burs

tive materials have all played a part in this revolution. Some carious lesions may now be monitored if they are judged to be arrested or inactive. Cavities are now kept much smaller and the maximum amount of sound tooth substance is maintained.

During cavity preparation all high-speed rotating engine instruments require that a water spray is used to cool the cut tooth surface during the operation. The DSA may be required to control the air and water sprays, and aspirate water and debris during the treatment, maintaining clear visibility of the tooth and protecting the patient's airway. This procedure generally follows the same sequence:

1. *The outline form.* (This is now governed by the extent of the caries rather than a preconceived design.) Access is gained to the caries and the cavity is extended to eliminate caries wherever it occurs at the enamel–dentine junction in this particular tooth. All carious or unsupported enamel is removed.
2. *The convenience form.* The cavity may have to be opened further to allow instrumentation. The cavity margins are planned so that they are in the best position for appearance, and for future cleaning and assessment.
3. *The resistance form* is developed so that the final restoration and the remaining tooth substance will be able to withstand masticatory pressures.
4. *The retention form* takes into account the restorative material that is to be used. The cavity is shaped to ensure that the restoration will be held firmly in place.
5. All remaining caries is removed.
6. The margins of the cavity are smoothed and finished carefully.
7. All debris is removed from the cavity.

Temporary restorations

After the cavity preparation has been completed it may not be convenient or advisable to fill the tooth permanently at the same sitting in which case the tooth is dressed with a temporary filling. This must be non-irritant or even have a sedative effect, it should be quick-setting, firm when set, resistant to masticatory pressure, able to stabilize the tooth, and yet easily removed when necessary.

Common temporary dressings include stiffly mixed zinc oxide and eugenol paste, accelerated zinc oxide/eugenol (with zinc acetate as the accelerator), zinc phosphate cement and zinc polycarboxylate cement.

CAVITY LININGS

Before any permanent restoration is placed on top of a cut and prepared dentine surface a lining must be considered. Linings may be considered to have therapeutic and structural properties. Lining materials will protect the pulp from thermal or chemical influences during and after the introduction of the filling material, they prevent micro-leakages, and they can do much to support the tooth and restore the internal shape of the cavity. By covering the dentinal surface in this way internal staining of the tooth by amalgam is prevented.

Very deep cavities may be sublined with a calcium hydroxide cement to encourage the formation of secondary dentine in the pulp. Other lining cements are chosen because they are easy to manipulate, adhere to the walls of the cavity and set quickly enough for the final restoration to be packed upon them immediately without any possibility of the lining being displaced or crushed.

Common lining cements include resin-reinforced quick-setting zinc oxide/eugenol, zinc polycarboxylate and zinc phosphate.

Varnishes are sometimes used in prepared cavities, for example, to protect dentine from chemical irritants or to improve the marginal sealing of amalgam.

Mixing reinforced zinc oxide/eugenol cement
This is *not* a suitable lining for composite materials.

1. Portions of the white powder and yellow liquid are set out on a glass or paper slab, powder to liquid ratio 4:1.
2. With a metal spatula the powder and liquid are mixed together, in 1 minute, to form a stiff paste.
3. The paste will set in about 5 minutes.
4. Plastic instruments can be dipped into plain powder to prevent the cement from sticking to them.

Mixing zinc polycarboxylate cement
This sticks to both enamel and stainless steel.

1. Mix, according to the manufacturer's instructions, on a paper slab using a steel spatula, to form a stiff paste.
2. The material should be used immediately or it will become 'cobwebby'.
3. Clean the spatula at once with a wet gauze.
4. The material sets in about 5 minutes.

Mixing zinc phosphate cement
1. Portions of the cement powder and liquid are placed on a cold glass mixing slab. The liquid bottle must not be left open to the air for any longer than necessary or the water content will change and this will upset the properties of the cement and its setting times in future mixes.
2. The powder is divided into smaller portions with a metal mixing spatula.

3. Each small portion of cement powder is added to the liquid and thoroughly spatulated (mixed in) before the next portion is incorporated. The more slowly the first portions are added to the liquid, the longer the final setting time will be.
4. The whole mass is thoroughly mixed to incorporate as much powder as possible, to increase its strength and also to reduce its acid effect on the dentine and pulp.
5. The thick mix is transferred to the dried cavity and shaped with appropriate plastic instruments. To prevent the cement from sticking to the instruments they may be dipped in a small pile of dry cement powder or alcohol.

MATRICES

Where the cavity outline extends over more than a single surface of the tooth the final restoration material generally has to be packed into a box shape with one wall missing. In order to contain the filling material and allow it to be condensed properly a fourth wall has to be constructed temporarily as a matrix or shaper.

Types of matrix

Metal. A piece of thin stainless steel strip is held around the circumference of the tooth by a matrix holder or clamp. The band has to be held firmly against the tooth with wedges at the cervical margin in class II cavities to prevent the filling material from extruding under packing pressure. Many different patterns of matrix holders are available such as the Siqueland and Tofflemire.

Plastic. Thin plastic matrix strip is used to support most anterior filling materials, while they are being packed, held in place by the operator's fingers or with wedges and composition. Their transparency allows the operator to judge the position of the filling and any excess material at the cavity margins without having to disturb the matrix. Cellulose acetate, celluloid or polyester strips are used, but the latter reacts chemically with polymerizing acrylic resin type materials.

Contoured matrices. Specially curved and shaped matrices can cope with particular problems such as the cervical margin or incisal edge restoration.

Plastic crown forms. Thin transparent crown forms are made in cellulose acetate and are used to control larger amounts of plastic restorative material, for example, in the construction of temporary crowns, and for acid-etch restorations of broken teeth.

Registers or matrix impressions. Before the cavity is cut a piece of heat-softened composition is pressed over the tooth to record its shape and the margins of the adjacent teeth. This register, suitably protected with thin tinfoil or acetate sheet, can be used to form and support the final plastic filling material and thus ensure a true restoration of shape.

In another method a preoperative alginate impression of the arch is taken and later used as the matrix for temporary restorations following extensive tooth preparation.

MIXING AND INSERTION OF THE FILLING MATERIAL

Plastic filling materials are soft and mouldable while they are being manipulated and packed into the prepared cavity in the tooth and then, within a short period of time, they harden and become resistant to displacement or fracture. Figure 8/8 illustrates some of the instruments used in filling prepared cavities.

Several different types of plastic filling materials are available. The commonest are silver amalgam and composite resins. The DSA should be familiar with the manufacturer's instructions for mixing the various filling materials which are in use in her particular practice.

Amalgam

Silver amalgam is an almost universal filling material that can be used in any class of cavity. It is not often used in the front of the mouth for aesthetic reasons. It is prepared by mixing together amalgam alloy (containing silver and tin with traces of copper and zinc), in a finely powdered form, with clean mercury. Amalgam alloy is now available as lathe-cut particles or spherical particles. The latter makes a more fluid mix of amalgam. Amalgam is mixed and used in the following manner:

1. The proportion of alloy powder and mercury must be accurately dispensed by weight or other measuring system. Too much mercury causes the amalgam to expand excessively and reduces its flow and strength; too little mercury causes loss of working properties and porosity. A ratio of 1 part of alloy to 1.6 parts of mercury by weight is generally found to be the most suitable though the manufacturer's directions should be followed carefully.
2. Amalgam is never mixed by hand because of the dangers of mercury poisoning. It is mixed:
   a. In sealed capsules from the manufacturer used in an automatic vibrator;
   b. In an enclosed amalgamator machine which internally doses out the mercury and alloy into a mixing chamber. The proportions of the mix

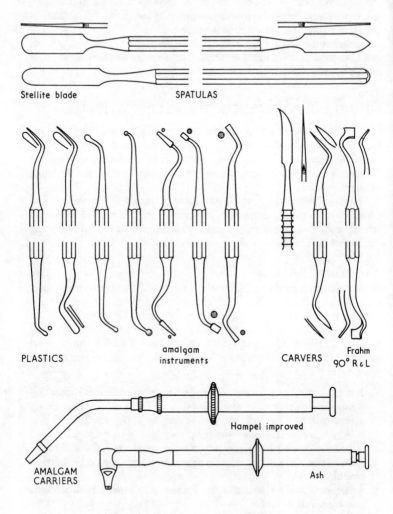

Stellite blade   SPATULAS

PLASTICS   amalgam instruments   CARVERS   Frahm 90° R & L

AMALGAM CARRIERS   Hampel improved   Ash

Fig. 8/8 Spatulas, plastics, carvers and amalgam carriers

are adjustable. The machine has to be refilled from stock containers from time to time;

c. The alloy and mercury are dispensed by hand into reusable capsules which are then mixed in a vibrator.

In all cases the soft amalgam mix will have a smooth, silvery appearance. Excessive mixing breaks down the crystal structure.

3. Small portions of the amalgam are conveyed to the dried cavity in an amalgam carrier and condensed into place with maximum pressure using serrated amalgam pluggers or a mechanical engine condenser to bring excess mercury to the surface (Fig. 8/9).

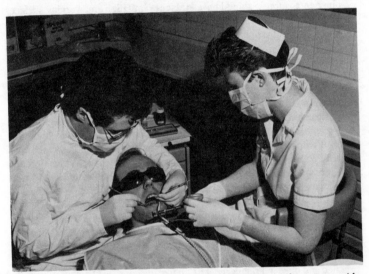

Fig. 8/9 Packing an amalgam restoration. The DSA is presenting the operator with further amalgam

4. Subsequent portions of amalgam are added to the first and condensed into place until the cavity is overfilled.

5. After the filling has hardened the excess material, which contains the surplus mercury, is cut away with carving instruments, any matrix is removed and the restoration is contoured to shape.

6. The restoration is checked for height of bite and general occlusion, adjusted as necessary by further carving and may then be smoothed with moist cottonwool pellets.

7. Before he is dismissed the patient is warned to avoid heavy pressure or eating upon the restored tooth for at least an hour.

Health and safety note regarding the use of mercury

Mercury is poisonous. It can be *absorbed through the skin* and the hands should be washed immediately after handling anything that contaminates them with metallic mercury. At room temperature mercury vaporizes into the air and can be *absorbed by inhalation*. Eating, drinking, smoking and the application of cosmetics should not be allowed in the dental surgery because of the dangers of *absorption by swallowing* from mercury-contaminated hands and the environment. (Once the amalgam has set in the tooth all free mercury is fixed chemically and cannot poison the patient.)

The dental surgery should have efficient ventilation and working surfaces and floors should have hard, smooth surfaces with the minimum of crevices in which spilled mercury droplets could collect. Cleaning equipment and mops used on the surgery floor should not be used in other areas of the practice. A domestic vacuum cleaner must *never* be used in the dental surgery for this will rapidly raise the mercury vapour levels in the air.

All manipulations of mercury (for example, mixing amalgam or transferring mercury from one container to another) should be carried out over a drip tray. All mercury, waste amalgam and other residues should be stored in well-sealed, non-metallic containers in a cool place. Waste should be covered with water in its collecting container to trap vapour. Waste must never be washed down the sink or left in a general wastebin. Waste mercury, amalgam and recovered spillage is valuable and when sufficient has accumulated it can be returned to the supplier for recovery.

Mercury spillage. Should mercury be spilt accidentally the dental surgeon must be informed immediately. Under his direction every effort must be made to recover every particle of the spilt mercury or to render it harmless. Equipment for dealing with spillage should be readily available in the practice and checked regularly. The kit usually consists of disposable plastic gloves, paper towels, a rubber bulb aspirator to draw up large globules of mercury, a container into which the mercury and contaminated items can be collected and sealed and a mercury absorbent paste (composed of equal parts of flowers of sulphur and hydrated calcium hydroxide, moistened with water) or a special proprietary substance for this purpose. After dealing with the spillage the room must be aired thoroughly via an open window.

Glass ionomer cements (GIC)

These materials adhere to both dentine and enamel and can leach (wash out a soluble component) fluoride at the cavity margins. They are very useful for restoring class V cervical cavities. They are very water-sensitive and need to be varnished during the hardening period to prevent the movement of water in or out of the material.

Debris and grease are cleaned from the surface of the dentine with 50 per cent citric acid, subsequently washed off, before the cement is applied to the dried surface. Thus deep cavities must be protected with calcium hydroxide base. These cements should be mixed according to their manufacturer's instructions using an abrasion-resistant spatula. Mixed in 1 minute, they set in 3 minutes and become extremely hard in 5 minutes. GIC Cermets (such as Ketac-silver) incorporate silver/glass particles and can be used to build up strong cores in teeth.

Composite filling materials

These expensive materials consist of special resins which have up to 80 per cent of other materials added to them to improve their hardness, appearance and working properties. Such a resin differs from ordinary acrylic resin (it may be the reaction product of an epoxy resin with methacrylic acid). The additives may be tiny glass beads or rods, particles of quartz or lithium aluminium silicate. Unopened packets should be stored under refrigeration to extend shelf-life.

The shade and translucency of the basic material can be altered at the chairside when required by the addition of special colouring agents.

These materials are mainly used in class III, IV and V restorations and, using the acid etch technique, in veneering and restoring stained, malformed or fractured teeth, periodontal splinting and orthodontic bonding. Recently new composites have been developed for use in posterior teeth.

For restorations.
1. The tooth is cleaned with an oil-free, non-fluoride polishing paste and rinsed thoroughly.
2. The cavity is prepared.
3. The tooth is isolated and dried.
4. The exposed dentine surfaces are lined and protected with an eugenol-free material such as a calcium hydroxide base.
5. The enamel walls of the cavity are etched with an acid solution, applied with a cotton-wool pledget, for 60 seconds. (Enamel on primary teeth requires 2 minutes' etching.)
6. The tooth is washed thoroughly with a water spray. (The patient must not rinse out or the etched surface will be contaminated with saliva.)
7. The tooth is isolated and dried thoroughly, when the etched surface will have a white frosty appearance.
8. The bonding layer is applied according to the manufacturer's instructions.
9. The restorative filled resin is placed over the bond layer.

Chemically activated resins are mixed from two component pastes on a paper slab. The cavity is filled immediately and the material controlled with a matrix or crown form while it is setting.

Light-activated resins are presented ready-mixed in lightproof containers. A small quantity is dispensed on to a paper slab (which can still be shielded from light with a plastic lid) and used to fill the cavity in incrementally cured layers which allow the operator greater control over the shape and colour of the restoration. This material is 'light-cured' when activated by an intense light from a special source delivered by a fibreoptic cable. *Note*: it is important not to stare at this bright light, for it can damage the eyes. Special orange protective glasses or shields are available.

10. Any hard excess material is removed with rotating diamond instruments, but the best results are obtained if such reduction can be kept to a minimum and the 'matrix shine' can be retained. (See also the acid etch technique of restoring broken teeth described on page 191.)

Note: Any acid accidentally contacting oral tissues, eyes or skin should *immediately* be flushed away with copious amounts of water. Uncovered etched enamel surfaces recover their normal appearance in a few days.

Retention pins

All plastic filling materials can be given better retention and reinforcement where necessary by the use of special metal pins. Basically, these are made of inert, threaded wire cut to an appropriate short length and, if necessary, bent into shape. The pins are cemented or threaded into prepared pinholes that have been drilled into the periphery of the cavity, away from the pulp, using special fine pinhole burs of the same diameter as the pin wire; self-tapping pins are also available.

FINISHING AND POLISHING

Amalgam (after 48 hours)

1. The surface is smoothed with engine-driven stones, finishing burs and sandpaper discs.
2. The interproximal surfaces are polished with linen polishing strips by hand.
3. The whole surface is polished with pumice powder and water paste on engine-driven rubber cups and bristle brushes.
4. The final polish is completed with a whiting and alcohol paste applied with a clean, soft brush, rotating at high speed and light pressure.

Composite filling materials and GIC (after the recommended time)

1. Any bulk excess is removed with chisels or sharp scalpel blades.

2. Further contouring or reduction is carried out with rotating fine-diamond stones or special burs, sometimes lubricated with petroleum jelly.
3. The surface may be smoothed, if necessary, with white mounted stone points and composite finishing points, followed by various grades of polishing discs and interproximal strips.

CHAPTER NINE

Inlays, Crowns and Bridgework

In addition to the plastic restoration techniques in which the materials are packed, moulded, allowed to harden and finished in the prepared tooth, other restorations can be fabricated outside the mouth on models and then cemented into place. Care and precision and the highest standards of work are necessary if this complex type of treatment is to meet with success.

INLAYS

An inlay is a cast gold restoration shaped to fit accurately into a cavity prepared in the crown of a tooth. They are used most commonly to restore badly broken down posterior teeth that have to withstand considerable masticatory pressure or to support bridges.

In general an inlay cavity when prepared and lined must have retentive, almost parallel walls without any undercuts, sharp internal cavity angles and should have a flat seating floor. Where appropriate the enamel margins at the cavo-surface angle around the periphery of the cavity are bevelled, for example, at the occlusal and gingival margins. This will remove weakened enamel prisms and also improve the marginal fit of the final restoration, because gold has a good edge strength and 'feather-edge' produced can be burnished in this region. The main retention of the finished inlay comes from its overall sliding fit into the cavity assisted by the grip and locking effect of the final cementing medium. The line of withdrawal should, when possible, be in the line of, and in the opposite direction to the stresses likely to be placed upon it in the mouth. Still further retention can be obtained when necessary by the use of pins and ridges cast onto the basic inlay that will fit into prepared pinholes (Fig. 9/2) and slots cut into the tooth.

Basically, inlay preparations can be described using Black's classification although it is unusual to construct class I inlays in occlusal surfaces. Modern dentistry finds little indication for simple inlays (Fig. 9/1), and the method now tends to be reserved for cases where the cusps of the tooth are undermined, weakened or lost and full cuspal coverage or replacement with gold is required. In situations where a minimal amount of tooth needs to be removed interproximally a 'slice-preparation' is used (see Fig. 9/2).

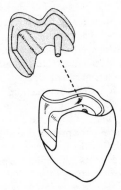

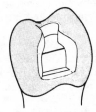

Fig. 9/1 Class II gold inlay cavity on a premolar

Fig. 9/2 Class II inlay preparations in a premolar. Note the retention pin

IMPRESSION TECHNIQUES

Direct impressions
A piece of inlay wax is heated in a flame, pressed into the prepared cavity, cooled and then trimmed and contoured to the correct shape and occlusion. In complex cavities the inlay wax may have to be controlled in the first instance with a metal matrix band positioned around the tooth. Once the pattern has been satisfactorily prepared it may be removed from the cavity with a probe or sprue, taking care not to bend or distort the wax. The wire sprue is heated and attached to the pattern at its thickest point, well away from its edges or fitting surface, before sending it to the laboratory for immediate investment and casting (see Laboratory Technique, p. 122). This technique requires special skill, can really only be used for very simple inlays which then require time-consuming polishing in the mouth, and is mainly superseded by the indirect methods.

Indirect impressions
This is the best method for making complex multi-surface inlays particularly in inaccessible regions of the mouth. An accurate impression of the cavity and adjacent teeth is taken, together with a record of the shape of the opposing teeth and registration of occlusion. Models are then prepared in the laboratory, mounted in articulation, and the inlay is constructed on them. This method demands special care in the impression and model-making stages to ensure that small inaccuracies cannot occur that will spoil the fit of the finished inlay.

Elastic impressions. Various non-reversible elastic impression materials are available that are based on mercaptan or silicone rubbers. These materials are creamy when mixed, but set into a tough, stable, rubbery and elastic consistency that will give extremely accurate detailed impressions of inlay and crown preparations and the adjacent teeth and tissues. They can reproduce undercuts. Using these materials and a careful technique, several inlay cavities may be prepared in the same quadrant of the mouth at once and, with a single impression, all the inlays completed and fitted at the second appointment.

These materials require a special tray. Before taking the impression the quadrant with the prepared teeth is dried and isolated. The gingival margins next to the cavities may need to be retracted with an astringent packing string (removed before impression) to prevent oozing and to allow the paste to flow into place.

Rubber base. This material is usually dark brown and has a characteristic smell. The special tray must be coated with a tray adhesive. The material is usually of two sorts: light and heavy-bodied. The light-bodied material is flowed over the preparations, sometimes with a special syringe, and then the tray filled with the heavy-bodied material carried into place. These materials are slow-setting – an advantage with multiple preparations. They are usually presented as two pastes which are mixed together with a spatula on a large paper slab.

Silicone rubber.
1. *Condensation-curing silicones.* These early materials are used in a two-stage impression method in which a correcting 'wash' of thin material is added to a set preliminary impression which is then replaced in the mouth. This technique can lead to distortion of the final impression. The set impression will soon shrink and must be cast immediately.
2. *Addition-curing silicones.* These new materials are very accurate and stable. They do not flow easily over the preparations. They are used in a special tray in a putty and wash method with both materials setting in the mouth together. The set impression should not be cast immediately to allow gases to escape from the material.

Temporary restorations
These are very important to protect the tooth, stabilize its position and prevent gingival overgrowth during the period of inlay construction. The material used must be easily and cleanly removable at the next appointment.

LABORATORY TECHNIQUE

Briefly, the impression must be cast into accurate, hard, working models. The prepared tooth model may be cast individually in extra-hard stone or produced by copper plating. The resultant tooth model or die is then seated into the larger impression of the arch and the whole model can then be cast up and articulated with the model of the opposing teeth. Some operators prefer that the model should be cast in one stage to avoid seating errors of such precast dies.

The inlay pattern is waxed up on the die, sprued with a length of wire and removed from the model. At this stage, both the direct wax and the indirect proceed in the same way (Fig. 9/3).

The wax pattern to be cast is coated with a layer of semiliquid investment material which is similar in consistency to dental plaster. The coated pattern is then set in a metal casting ring and surrounded by further investment material. Great care must be taken to avoid air bubbles in the investment that would spoil the final casting, and these are eliminated by vibration or vacuum techniques.

When the investment has set, the sprue is removed and the ring and its contents heated in a furnace. The wax melts and burns away leaving a space into which molten gold can be cast.

The casting is then cleaned, polished, fitted to the model and returned to the surgery.

FITTING AND CEMENTING THE INLAY

The temporary dressing is removed from the cavity and the inlay tried in to check the fit, the margins, the bite height and the contact points with the adjacent teeth. Any minor adjustments can be made at the chairside and the gold repolished, but with an accurate technique and careful work in the laboratory this should rarely be necessary. The gold margins are burnished carefully to ensure that they are perfectly adapted to the tooth surface. The inlay is washed in alcohol to remove any grease from polishing or handling it and dried. The cavity is washed and the tooth isolated with cottonwool rolls and saliva ejector and dried with a jet of warm air. A thin mix of zinc phosphate or other luting cement is prepared and some is coated over the fitting surface of the inlay before more is carried to the tooth surface with an instrument. Thus the higher temperature of the tooth, which accelerates the cement setting time, will not be a problem. The inlay is placed in position in the mouth and pressed well home with an instrument. Some dental surgeons like to tap the inlay home with an automatic mallet. If necessary the inlay may be held in place by getting the patient to bite on a wood point (the kind used for interdental cleansing) positioned over the inlay. When the cement has set, the extruded excess is removed from all the margins and between the teeth with a probe and floss silk. The result should be an inlay with its margins in firm accurate contact with the tooth and no cement line.

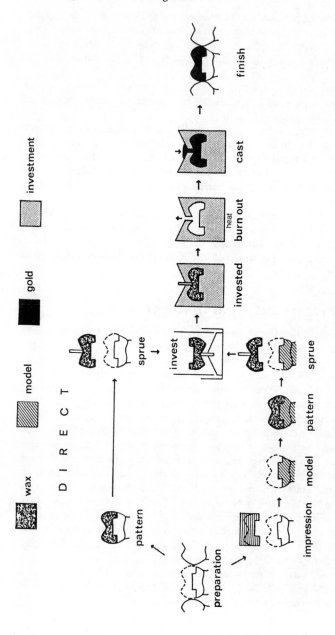

Fig. 9/3 The laboratory stages of making an inlay by direct and indirect methods

PORCELAIN VENEERS

Discoloured, misshapen teeth can be improved aesthetically with a minimum of preparation by covering the labial surface with a porcelain veneer. The tooth enamel is reduced minimally to make room for the 0.5–0.7mm thick facing and a silicone impression taken. Temporary cover, though rarely needed, can be provided by a layer of composite on unetched enamel. The fit surface of the veneer is acid-etched and then treated with a special silene coupling agent in the laboratory. This agent bonds the porcelain to the composite used to attach the veneer to the acid-etched tooth.

CROWNS

A crown is a very extensive restoration of the coronal structure of a tooth and may be prepared on anterior or posterior teeth. Crowns are classified according to their design or the material of which they are made.

Jacket crowns

These are generally used on anterior teeth for they can give a very good aesthetic appearance.

Porcelain. See Fig. 9/4. The whole enamel surface of the tooth is removed with diamond instruments to leave a dentine peg protecting the pulp, and a cervical shoulder is prepared. A full impression in rubber is taken as for an inlay together with an alginate impression of the opposing teeth and an accurate colour shade record. In the laboratory the porcelain crown is constructed by fusing together tinted porcelain powders on a die-prepared

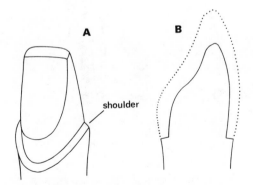

Fig. 9/4 A. Incisor prepared for a porcelain jacket crown
B. Lateral aspect to show outline of the finished crown

platinum matrix in a special furnace and finally glazing the surface. The platinum lining the finished crown must be removed before it is cemented into place. Very accurate and detailed colour matches can be obtained and the slightly translucent porcelain looks exactly like natural enamel.

Porcelain bonded to gold. In this method the preparation needs a wider labial shoulder than for a porcelain jacket crown, but does not require a wide cervical shoulder on the palatal or interproximal surface because these regions of the crown are covered with a veneer of gold. Porcelain is heat bonded to the labial and incisal surfaces of the gold to give a good aesthetic result. (Acrylic may also be used in this way but is less resistant to wear and not as colour-fast.)

Post crowns
When all the coronal structure of the tooth is lost, or the tooth weakened by root canal therapy or very extensive caries, any crown has to be made on a central reinforcing post or post and core.

Post or dowel crown. The natural crown is removed to gingival level and the root canal cleaned of filling to an adequate depth to hold the post. The surface of the remaining tooth substance is prepared to support the crown and prevent it from rotating. In one of several possible techniques an impression of both the prepared root face and the root canal may be taken together. The usual locating impressions, bite and tooth shade are required.

Post and core. In this method the post is made first and cemented into place before the crown is constructed (Fig. 9/5). After preparing the canal as

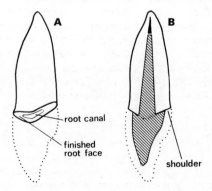

Fig. 9/5 A. Incisor ready for gold post and core
B. Gold post and core fitted and prepared for a porcelain jacket crown.
The tooth has been apically sealed

before, a wire of wrought gold or other suitable metal is waxed up as necessary to fit the canal and to produce a coronal extension similar in shape to the final crown preparation. Additional gold is cast on to the wire in the laboratory and the post and core cemented into place. A conventional full crown preparation is made and a jacket crown constructed and cemented into place.

Three-quarter crowns
These are really extensive veneer gold inlays used to reinforce weakened teeth or to make a firm abutment for a bridge. Three-quarter of the surface of the tooth may be removed in this preparation (Fig. 9/6), together with the

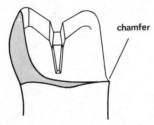

Fig. 9/6 Three-quarter crown preparation on a molar from the mesial aspect

incisal edge or the occlusal surface, but commonly leaving the buccal or labial enamel untouched for appearance. Retention is gained with inter-proximal slots or pins placed so that the final crown is inserted from the incisal or occlusal direction. Ideally, retention grooves should be placed as far buccally as possible to achieve the greatest length and effect. (The chamfer or bevelled shoulder is becoming less popular because its feather edge may lead to wax distortion and casting defects in this region.)

Full crowns
Badly broken down posterior teeth can be restored with full gold crowns covering all clinical surfaces (Fig. 9/7). The preparations can be shoulder-less or to a shoulder. Full crowns of this kind can be constructed on pinned amalgam cores for badly destroyed teeth and will do much to support weakened enamel and dentine by giving *extracoronal retention* around the outside of the tooth. The impression technique is broadly that described for indirect inlays.

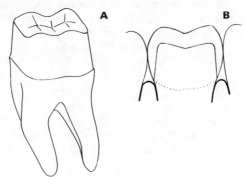

Fig. 9/7 A. Full veneer crown preparation on a molar from the mesial aspect
B. Section from the buccal aspect with tooth in situ and crown fitted

Temporary crown restorations

These are very important for aesthetic reasons, to protect and stabilize the tooth and also to hold back the gingival margins.

Temporary crowns may be constructed of acrylic in the laboratory to impressions taken before the preparations are made, they may be made with preformed crown forms filled with acrylic or other plastic (for example, Scutan) at the chairside, or from cold-cure acrylic materials shaped between the prepared tooth and a prepreparation alginate impression. The crowns are fixed with temporary cement. Posterior teeth can also be protected with selected and marginally trimmed aluminium crown forms filled with quick-setting zinc oxide cement.

Fitting and cementing the crown

The technique is similar to that used for an inlay. The margins, occlusion, overall contour, contact points, shade and general appearance are checked, and for anterior crowns the patient should also be allowed to examine and approve the appearance before the crown is finally cemented into place with zinc phosphate cement.

BRIDGES

Dental bridges are non-removable appliances constructed to restore a missing tooth or teeth and attached to the adjacent sound teeth. They may be based on:

1. Foundation teeth prepared for crowns, *abutments*, to support the span of the bridge, the *pontic*;
2. More recently, on minimal preparations.

Bridge pontics may be rigidly fixed to the abutment at each end, *fixed-fixed*, or they may have an interlocking attachment at one end that allows a little independent movement between the abutment teeth, *fixed-movable* (Fig. 9/8.) Prefabricated precision attachments are available to help in planning and constructing the movable attachment.

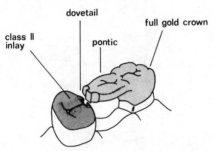

Fig. 9/8 A fixed-movable bridge with sanitary pontic filling saddle area in the position of the first molar

Assessment and design
Before a bridge can be constructed the mouth has to be assessed clinically, as well as by study models and radiographs to check and consider such things as the periodontal health, the strength of the root attachments, the caries rate, the occlusion, the span of the proposed bridge, and so on, before a design can be made. Not every case is suitable.

Types of bridge preparation
Anterior bridges. These are usually constructed for aesthetic purposes to replace a lost tooth. All gold in the abutment teeth is kept as invisible as possible using tooth-coloured facings where necessary. The abutments may be inlays usually with full cuspal coverage, three-quarter crowns or full crowns depending upon the shape, position and condition of the supporting teeth. *Cantilever* bridges may be indicated in which a crown on a posterior tooth (for example, premolar or canine); supports an anterior tooth (for

example, a central incisor) on a firm gold bar curving forward and out of sight behind the teeth. This puts considerable strain and leverage on the posterior tooth. *Spring cantilever* bridges have a similar design but a more flexible gold bar is used that gains some support from the underlying mucosae (Fig. 9/9).

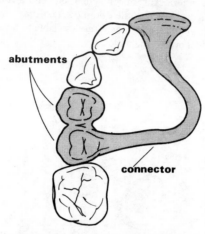

abutments

connector

Fig. 9/9 Spring cantilever bridge designed to replace missing central incisor. Full gold crowns on the premolars with a soldered joint between them act as the abutment

Posterior bridges. Here the main requirement is to provide a good masticatory surface for the opposing teeth to work against. Sturdy abutment teeth are essential and often full gold crowns are used. Where the aesthetic appearance is not important a *sanitary pontic* is used in which a space is left between the occlusal working surface and the mucosa to allow the tongue and normal oral hygiene methods better access for cleaning under the bridge (see Fig. 9/8).

Technique of bridge construction
1. Assess the case and plan the bridge.
2. Prepare the abutment teeth.
3. Take impressions of the abutment teeth.
4. Take the bite, shade and impression of the opposing teeth.
5. Place the temporary restorations.
6. Try in the abutment restorations.
7. Take a locating impression of the abutments.

8. Place further temporary restorations.
9. Try in the completed bridge.
10. Cement the bridge into place.
11. Show the patient how to clean the bridge properly.
12. Follow up at intervals to check function.

Minimal preparation bridges

The 'Maryland' or 'Rochette' bridge methods attach the pontic to the adjacent teeth via a metal framework retained on the enamel by composite and the acid-etch technique. The method is particularly useful for young patients who wish to avoid a removable denture. Minimal preparation is required to obtain a path of insertion (sometimes no preparation is necessary) and an elastic impression is taken for the laboratory. Retention for the framework is assisted in the Maryland bridge by etching the fit surface in the laboratory, and in the Rochette bridge undercut perforations are made in the fitting surfaces through which the attaching composite flows and locks.

CHAPTER TEN

Pulp Treatment and Root Canal Therapy

The restoration of teeth is often complicated by the proximity of the advancing carious process to the pulp. When the caries extends into the pulp chamber, acute or chronic inflammation, *pulpitis*, abscess or death of the pulp, *pulpal necrosis*, will occur and the infective process may proceed further to cause periapical infection. Sometimes, if the patient does not receive treatment, the pain and discomfort of this infective process can settle down to a painless chronic condition that no longer seems to him to require attention. Untreated dead teeth or chronic apical infection have long been regarded as a continual hazard to the patient's general health, particularly in cases with heart valve lesions, etc. By modern pulp treatment, root canal therapy (*endodontics*) and apical surgery techniques, infection and chronic apical inflammation can be eliminated in many cases, otherwise the affected tooth will have to be extracted.

CASE SELECTION

A non-vital tooth may be selected for pulp or root canal therapy in a cooperative patient who has no medical contraindications, whose general oral condition merits this treatment, where the tooth is of value for appearance, masticatory or denture or bridge support reasons and where the individual tooth's condition gives a good chance of success.

PULP DIAGNOSIS

1. Take a case history of any pain, noting its onset, intensity and duration.
2. Make a clinical examination noting any cavity, fracture, local apical swelling, inflammation or sinus, tenderness to percussion or looseness in the socket.
3. Special tests:
   a. Pulp vitality tests with heat (hot gutta percha) and cold (ice or evaporating ethyl chloride on cottonwool) or with the electric pulp tester.

  b. Radiographic examination to observe the depth of the cavity, the anatomy of the root canal and the periapical condition.
  c. Excavation of the cavity to see if there is an opening into the pulp chamber (pulp exposure).

TREATMENT METHODS

Pulpitis

Painful inflammation of the unexposed pulp can sometimes be resolved in its earliest stages by removing the cause (exposed dentine, caries, chemical or thermal irritants) and filling the cavity with a sedative dressing, such as zinc oxide and eugenol paste, for a few days.

Pulp capping

This is carried out on a vital tooth where a small, non-infected exposure of the pulp has occurred. The exposure is covered with a calcium hydroxide paste that will encourage the formation of secondary dentine to seal the breach and maintain the vitality of the pulp. The tooth is filled permanently and tested at intervals in later months to ensure that the pulp remains healthy.

Pulpotomy

When the exposure is large and potentially infected the crown pulp is removed under anaesthesia and sterile conditions leaving vital, non-infected pulp tissue undisturbed in the root canal. In young patients this may allow an unformed tooth apex to continue to grow normally. The amputated surface is covered with calcium hydroxide paste and the tooth filled permanently. It should be kept under regular radiographic survey in case the tooth requires conventional root treatment subsequently.

Pulpectomy

When the whole pulp is infected it becomes necessary to remove the total contents of the pulp chamber both in the crown and root or roots. The tooth is anaesthetized if necessary and then isolated with rubber dam and a good saliva ejector. The surface of the tooth is cleaned with a disinfectant solution and the tooth is opened with sterile burs. Once access to the root canal is gained the pulp is removed with a fine barbed broach passed up into the canal and rotated to catch and hold the pulp tissue.

Drainage

When pulpal inflammation has proceeded to pus formation some periapical swelling and infection may occur. In these circumstances it may be necessary to leave the tooth open to drain away the pus and inflammatory exudates for 24 hours or so before the root canal therapy can be continued. With severe infections general supportive treatment and antiobiotics may be indicated.

Measurement of root canal length
An accurate determination of the length of a root canal can be made by taking a radiograph of it while a metal root canal instrument of known length lies inside the tooth. By measuring the apparent length of the known instrument and the apparent length of the unknown root canal on the radiograph, the working length of the root canal can be calculated by simple proportion.

Preparation of the root canal
The canal has to be cleaned to eliminate infected dentine, enlarged, all debris removed and the canal rendered sterile before a permanent root filling can be put into it.

Instrumentation. The walls of the root canal are cleaned and prepared using reamers and files (Fig. 10/1).

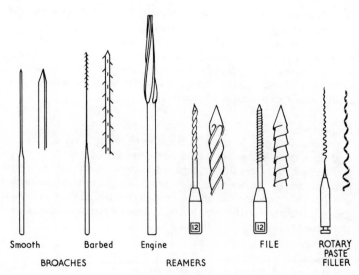

| Smooth | Barbed | Engine | | FILE | ROTARY PASTE FILLER |
| BROACHES | | REAMERS | | | |

Fig. 10/1 Some examples of endodontic instruments

Reamers are gently rotated in the root canal by thumb and finger action. Special handpieces are available which can oscillate instruments back and forth through a quadrant of movement. Great care has to be taken to avoid instrument fracture or perforation of the wall or apex of the canal.

Their spiral cutting action tends to work debris downwards towards the coronal end of the root canal.

Root canal files have serrated surfaces and are inserted into the root canal, pressed against one wall at a time and scraped out again to remove debris.

Sets of reamers and files are graded in diameter sizes and are used in an ascending sequence to gradually enlarge and prepare the root canal. These instruments are also made in various lengths to cope with teeth of different sizes. Measuring devices and adjustable stops on the instruments allow accurate working lengths to be achieved. Not every root canal can be penetrated completely for there may be mechanical problems due to curvatures or calcified blockages. Ideally the canal is reamed to a length 0.5mm short of the apex, a point of natural constriction in most mature teeth.

Asepsis. All root canals must be clean, dry and sterile before they are filled; infection must be eliminated for the patient's safety. Treatment is carried out using an aseptic technique with rubber dam in place to avoid contamination from the mouth. All instruments and materials used in the root canal must be sterile. Root canal therapy boxes may be made up containing all the instruments, cottonwool, paper points, etc., sterilized and kept immediately available for treatment. Infected debris is washed away from the canal with narrow-bore needles on a sterile syringe using sterile saline solution or dilute hydrogen peroxide solution followed by a solution of sodium hypochlorite. Fluid may be removed from the root canal with dry paper points which are absorbent. Disinfection of the canal is achieved by placing a paper point or cottonwool pledget in the tooth moistened with a disinfectant such as camphorated parachlorophenol and sealing it firmly into place for several days. Such a root canal dressing may have to be repeated at intervals until the canal is symptomless.

Filling the root canal

Once the canal has been prepared and sterilized it may be filled permanently (*obturated*) with a solid point of correct diameter and length, usually made of gutta percha or silver, sealed into place with a suitable cement. The walls of the canal are dried and then the canal is filled with a thin, creamy mix of slow-setting cement carried into place either by hand, using a reamer in reverse rotation, or with an engine-drive rotary paste filler (see Fig. 10/1). The core point is then carried up into place to its predetermined length. Additional accessory gutta percha points may be needed to pack laterally against the main point once it is in position. Finally, all the excess lengths of points still projecting from the cavity are cut off level with the opening of the canal and the cavity filled before removing the rubber dam. A check radiograph is taken immediately to confirm that the root filling is adequate, and the canal is filled to the apical constriction with no visible voids along its length.

Follow-up

All root-treated teeth are kept under routine clinical and radiographic observation to make sure that apical infection does not recur. Radiographs are taken at 3 months, 6 months and then annually for about 5 years to ensure that all is well.

Apical surgery

When apical infection cannot be permanently eradicated by root canal therapy, apical surgery will be necessary if the tooth is to be safely retained in the mouth. The infected apex is either scraped (*curetted*) or cut off and removed (*apicectomy*) and the apical granulation curetted away (see Oral Surgery, p. 166).

CHAPTER ELEVEN

Periodontology

Periodontology is the branch of dentistry concerned with the prevention and treatment of diseases involving the periodontal tissues. Periodontal disease, like dental caries, has an almost universal distribution throughout the human race and its incidence increases steadily with age. The real danger lies in the fact that it can cause slow, insidious and often painless deterioration of the supporting structures of the teeth which all too often remains unrecognized until treatment can no longer be effective and teeth are lost. Age-related surveys have shown that while dental caries is responsible for most of the extractions carried out in the first two decades of life, in later years the periodontal diseases become increasingly important. In the age-group 35–40 years they are responsible for more than 60 per cent of all extractions and this figure rises to over 80 per cent in people of 65 years and older. Early diagnosis is essential if treatment is to be effective, and it must be borne in mind that the first stages of disease can often be detected in adolescence.

PERIODONTAL DISEASE

This is the general term used to describe plaque-induced disease of the periodonteum, that is, the supporting tissues of the teeth (the cementum, the periodontal membrane, the alveolar bone and the overlying gingival tissues), and it can range in intensity from gingivitis to periodontosis.

Gingivitis

This is inflammation of the gingival tissues and is usually the first stage in the onset of periodontal disease. It may arise from a variety of local and general causes.

Local causes. The common local causes are all conditions that lead to poor oral hygiene and subsequent plaque accumulation leading to a constant irritation of the gingivae:

1. Inefficient tooth brushing and food stagnation.
2. A consistently soft diet that does nothing to stimulate and harden the gingival tissues.

3. Heavy tobacco smoking which tends to be associated with poor oral hygiene.
4. Irregularly arranged teeth, traumatic bites or unopposed teeth.
5. Untreated dental caries or inadequate or badly contoured restorations.
6. Ill-fitting dentures or orthodontic appliances.
7. Drying due to mouth-breathing.

Gingivitis is thus associated with the presence of plaque and calculus on the teeth and in the gingival crevice.

Plaque. Where oral hygiene is poor, dental plaque can build up rapidly in the gingival crevice. The plaque contains certain components which cause dental caries, and others which initiate periodontal disease. The products of this plaque are very irritant to the gingivae, causing inflammation and degeneration of the deeper tissues with irreversible breakdown and pocket formation. The deeper layers of established plaque can mineralize to form calculus.

Plaque index. There are several methods of scoring the extent of plaque present on the teeth. One is based on calculating a simple percentage of the number of tooth surfaces with plaque present, against the number of tooth surfaces available. Each tooth is scored as having four surfaces thus excluding the occlusal.

Calculus (tartar). This is commonly found in association with gingivitis and periodontal disease. It is a soft, yellow-white, porous material which hardens and stains with time. It can occur on teeth anywhere in the mouth but forms particularly on tooth surfaces that lie close to the openings of the salivary ducts: on the buccal sides of the maxillary molars opposite the paratoid ducts and on the lingual surface of the mandibular incisors opposite the sublingual ducts. Calculus is made up of about 70 per cent inorganic material and 30 per cent organic matter and water by weight. It is composed mainly of calcium phosphate and carbonate with traces of magnesium and other elements together with bacteria, epithelial cells and debris.

Supragingival calculus forms on the parts of the teeth that are visible above the gingival margin, and *subgingival calculus* forms just below the gingival margin.

When plaque and calculus are removed from the teeth the local gingival inflammation resolves in most cases – in other words, the condition is reversible.

General factors. There may also be general factors involved that predispose to gingivitis such as a vitamin deficiencies, blood disorders, hormonal changes, such as in pregnancy, and the use of certain drugs. It has also been reported that certain races are more susceptible to gingival diseases than others.

Acute inflammation of the gingival and periodontal tissues may be caused by local infections which are painful and require urgent treatment, for example, *acute ulcerative gingivitis* and *pericoronitis* which are discussed later, but generally gingival inflammation passes unnoticed into the chronic stage.

At first, in *chronic gingivitis*, the gingival margins are very slightly swollen and may bleed easily. If the disease is neglected the inflammation gradually spreads deeper to involve the periodontal membrane, etc. The condition may now be clinically termed chronic marginal periodontitis; the swollen gingivae become detached from the necks of the teeth and a true pocket is formed in which further food debris, plaque, calculus and inflammatory products can accumulate. This serious condition is usually painless and may also pass unnoticed by the patient although his near acquaintances will be aware that he has bad breath, *halitosis*.

Chronic periodontitis. Gradually, if untreated, the cementum becomes contaminated, the gingival attachment recedes towards the apical region of the tooth, the pockets enlarge, the fibres of the periodontal membrane are progressively destroyed, the gingivae recede and at the same time the alveolar bone of the socket is resorbed. This degree of loss of attachment is generally irreversible. Finally the tooth loosens and may be lost (See Fig. 3/3, p.59).

Diagnosis

A detailed case history is taken with particular attention to the patient's gingival symptoms (bleeding gums, loosening teeth, etc.), general health and medical and drug history. Special information is sought about the oral hygiene, dietary and smoking habits which all have a direct effect on the gingival and periodontal health.

The oral examination first records the general overall condition of the mouth, noting the oral hygiene, standard of conservation treatment and occlusion before proceeding to the detailed examination of the oral mucosa and teeth. A detailed record is made of the condition of the gingivae, the presence of calculus, the presence and extent of pocketing around the teeth, the mobility and occlusion of the individual teeth. The presence of dentures, bridgework or other appliances is noted. A specialized chart can be used to record the condition of the patient's periodontal structure by indicating the depth of pockets on a 2 mm horizontal line or grid system (see Fig. 6/2, p.88). The pocket depth can be measured accurately with a calibrated periodontal probe.

The Community Periodontal Index and Treatment Needs (CPITN) probe and scoring system (World Health Organization) uses the pocket depths of the most seriously affected tooth in each of the six sextants of the mouth (left, middle, right: upper and lower). The score obtained helps to decide clinical management of the case.

A radiograph examination to assess the alveolar bone loss follows, and models or bacteriological and blood tests may be required to complete the diagnosis.

TREATMENT

Initial preparation

This is aimed at eliminating as many of the causative factors as possible. It is essential that the patient deals with such matters as poor oral hygiene and attention to diet and general health. Acute conditions may require the use of antibiotics as well as local cleansing or even extraction to eliminate pain and infection. Once the condition of the mouth begins to improve, the results of previous neglect and damage can be tackled in the dental surgery.

Scaling and polishing

All plaque and calculus must be removed from the teeth if their irritant effects are to be overcome. Calculus, both supragingival and subgingival, is cleaned from the teeth by scaling. Scaling instruments are designed to be used to search out and remove calculus and to plane the tooth subgingivally to render its surface smooth. A very wide range of shapes of scalers is obtainable, but most dental surgeons confine themselves to a small number, perhaps half a dozen, that they personally find adequate for the purpose.

Scaling instruments (Fig. 11.1) fall into four main categories:

Supragingival scalers

Chisel or push scalers. These have a thin flexible end, tipped with a sharp blade, and are used to pass between the anterior teeth and dislodge calculus attached to their proximal surfaces.

Sickle scalers. These have blades that are triangular in cross-section and are used to remove supragingival calculus. The edge of the blade is carried below the gingival margin and the calculus is dislodged by pulling the instrument coronally while holding the blade firmly against the surface of the tooth.

Subgingival scalers

Hoe scalers. These are used mainly for the removal of subgingival calculus. The short blade projects at right angles to the shaft of the instrument. The tip

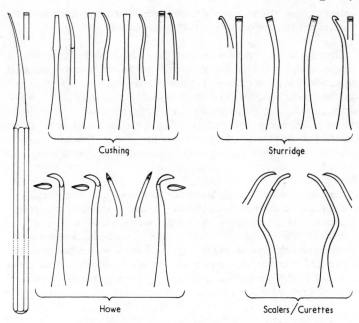

Cushing

Sturridge

Howe

Scalers / Curettes

Fig. 11/1 Some examples of scaling instruments

of the hoe is inserted into the pocket with the sharp surface towards the tooth, the calculus located by touch, the blade engaged and the material removed by a pull stroke.

Curettes. These are planing instruments, similar in shape to oval (cleiod) dentine excavators, used for removal of deep deposits of calculus and contaminated cementum.

All scaling instruments must be kept sharp, and to assist this some of the hoe scalers are made with extra-hard tungsten carbide tips.

Ultrasonic scalers. The apparatus can be separate or built into the dental unit, and has a lead to a special scaling handpiece. A sterilized insert with a scaler tip is placed into the handpiece and can be made to vibrate ultrasonically at 25 000 vibrations per second. The instrument will effectively remove calculus deposits from the teeth by both mechanical and ultrasonic activity. Several types of insert are available, each with a different action. Ultrasonic scaling is always carried out under a water spray for cooling and lavage. This requires efficient aspiration using high-speed suction.

After the scaling has been completed, polishing can be carried out to remove remaining stains and to smooth the tooth surfaces, and reduce their capacity to hold further plaque. The interdental surfaces are smoothed with fine linen polishing strips and dental floss coated in polishing paste. Finally, all the tooth surfaces are polished with a polishing paste using engine-driven rubber polishing cups and bristle brushes. A special handpiece should be used for polishing because the paste gets into the handpiece head and rapidly wears the moving parts spoiling them for accurate conservation work.

Root planing

In cases where there is established pocket formation, full mouth root planing will be required under local anaesthesia. The aim is to remove hard deposits and contaminated cementum from subgingival root surfaces.

After a further period of oral hygiene, carried out by the patient at home, considerable improvement in the gingival condition is the usual result and then a further assessment can be made of gingival contours and pockets to decide if further periodontal treatment, which may include periodontal surgery, is needed.

Gingival surgery

In suitable cases where the patient's cooperation, plaque control and interest is assured, moderate pockets can be eliminated surgically and the gingival contours can also be reshaped.

Surgery is carried out in stages so that the patient has only one side of the mouth operated upon at a time and can use the other comfortably during the healing stage.

Gingivectomy. This operation, once commonplace, is carried out less frequently now for it sacrifices gingival tissue and the end result may be unsightly. It is done mainly to remove enlarged soft tissue. Under anaesthesia the depths of the pockets in the operation site are marked (with the pocket-measuring forceps that punch through the pocket wall) to the level of the existing gingival attachment to the tooth. The unattached gingival tissue is then cut away by the use of specially angled gingivectomy knives (Fig. 11/2), such as Blake's Universal knife in which the tip of a Swann Morton scalpel blade is firmly held. The incision is carried along so that all the tissue is removed in one piece and afterwards any small tags remaining are carefully eliminated with further cautery or fine scissors. During the operation as in other forms of oral surgery, the DSA must work in close attendance using the sucker to keep the field free of saliva and blood.

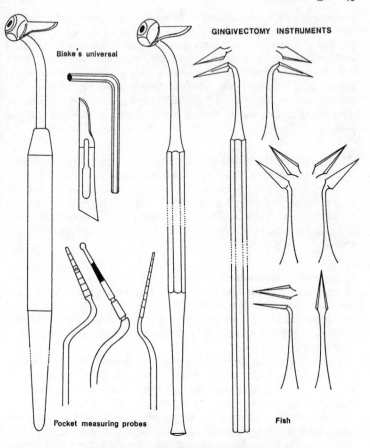

Blake's universal

GINGIVECTOMY INSTRUMENTS

Pocket measuring probes

Fish

Fig. II/2 Gingivectomy instruments

The wound is dressed with an antiseptic material such as Coe-Pack. The pack is applied to the wound from both the lingual and buccal or labial surface and pressed and moulded firmly into place. The patient is reviewed after a week.

Flap operations. These are carried out when it is necessary to gain access to the pockets and the underlying bone, for example, where bone defects exist as a result of periodontal disease and these have to be curetted (scraped) free of chronic infective products and granulation tissue to aid healing. When necessary the bone can be shaped and contoured with chisels or large sterile burs and diamond stones under a cooling stream of saline solution. The planned inverse bevel incision (to preserve gingival tissue) is made with a sharp scalpel with with a view to removing the epithelial lining of the pocket, and the tissue reflected from the bone with a periosteal elevator. All the undesirable material and calculus is removed and the surfaces of the teeth planed smooth. Then the flap is replaced and sutured into position. The operation area may be further protected with an antiseptic dressing pack.

After care. During the healing period, the patient is instructed to avoid eating on the operated side or disturbing the pack in any way. After about 7 days, the pack and sutures may be removed in the surgery and the patient must then keep the area clean with a soft toothbrush, and use a hot saline mouthwash for any soreness. As the area heals the patient can begin to brush the teeth and gingivae more vigorously each day and change to a medium toothbrush after about 2 to 3 weeks.

Functional abnormalities

In some cases the periodontal condition is aggravated by excessive occlusal pressures upon teeth due to malposition of a single tooth, malocclusion, premature loss of other teeth in the region, unopposed teeth, poor restorations, ill-fitting dentures or other appliances and nervous habits such as tooth-grinding (*bruxism*).

The occlusion is studied with the aid of models and by using articulating paper in the mouth to indicate points of contact. Treatment may be by selectively grinding away and reshaping certain teeth, by recontouring or replacing existing restorations, by remaking existing dentures or providing them for the first time so that they stabilize and support existing teeth. The effects of bruxism can be reduced by constructing a soft plastic bite guard, covering the occlusal surface of one jaw, to be worn by the patient at night.

In some cases, loosened teeth can be helped to survive occlusal pressures if they are splinted by a removable or fixed metal appliance to groups of healthy strong teeth elsewhere in the arch. Usually such matters are considered prior to the surgical phase.

Maintenance and prevention

Once the patient's course of treatment has been completed and his periodontal problem has been resolved as far as possible, it is vital that he is taught and maintains a high standard of oral hygiene (see page 201, Chapter 17) and returns every 3 to 6 months for thorough scaling and check-up.

Should a relapse occur the patient may once again be unable to detect it himself.

SPECIFIC INFLAMMATORY CONDITIONS

Acute ulcerative gingivitis (Vincent's disease)
The exact cause of this disease is obscure, but it always occurs in association with specific organisms: *B. fusiformis*, a non-motile, thin, curved organism with tapering ends, and *Borrelia vincenti*, a motile spirochaete. It is usually found in people of poor dental health, perhaps with a lowered general resistance to infection.

The onset of infection is sudden. Painful ragged ulcers occur locally on the interdental papillae and may spread quickly to affect the whole mouth and throat. There is a typical bad odour from the mouth, the temperature rises and the lymph nodes in the region are enlarged. The patient feels unwell and the appetite is lost.

Treatment. The mouth is gently cleansed with 10 volume hydrogen peroxide and peroxide mouthwashes are prescribed. At the same time a course of an antibiotic, such as penicillin, is given if the patient has a high temperature.

Metronidazole (Flagyl) is also used for oral Vincent's infection. The patient may need to take an analgesic, should avoid local irritation (smoking, hot spiced foods, etc.), ensure a high fluid intake and take plenty of rest. If necessary, investigation into the patient's general health is initiated. During the acute stage of the disease there is gross sepsis in the mouth and the patient should take common sense precautions to avoid contaminating his environment, for example, in the preparation of food. He should also throw away his old toothbrush and obtain a new one. When the acute stage has subsided attention should be given to necessary thorough scaling and other periodontal treatment, oral hygiene and general health and dietary considerations.

Acute herpetic stomatitis
This is a virus infection usually first affecting children under the age of six, and thought to be transmitted by direct contact when the virus gains access to the underlying tissues through a small breach in the epithelium of the mouth. (Stomatitis means inflammation of the mouth.)

Small vesicles or blisters develop on the oral mucosa or lips and then burst leaving an open, painful ulcer which rapidly becomes secondarily infected by other organisms. During an attack the temperature rises, the appetite falls and small children are distressed and unwell. The ulcers begin to heal in about seven days and are generally completely healed in 14 days. The herpes virus remains dormant in the healed tissues and can be reactivated in later years by changes in the local tissue environment, such as 'cold sores' on the lips.

Treatment. Drug therapy includes tetracycline mouthwashes, or the use of antiviral agents such as local idoxuridine or acyclovir (locally and systemically). Local symptoms may be eased by the application of topical anaesthetic and antiseptic ointments. The patient must be coaxed to take plenty of fluids and to eat cool, bland, non-spiced foods.

Pericoronitis

This is inflammation around an erupting tooth, generally a third molar, caused by eruption irritation, pressure on the overlying mucosa from the opposing tooth, food stagnation and secondary infection. The pain and discomfort is considerable and the patient may have swollen lymph nodes and find it difficult to open the mouth, *trismus*.

Treatment. This consists in raising the oral hygiene standards, the use of antiseptic mouthwashes, giving antibiotics if necessary and the removal of impacted teeth. In the acute stage extraction of the opposing tooth may be necessary.

Periodontal abscess

This is an abscess caused by spread of infection and destruction of tissue lateral to a tooth and deep in the periodontal tissues. Pus collects under pressure and there is localized painful swelling and inflammation below the gingival level. This condition must be differentiated from an apical abscess in which the infection arises as a result of a dead pulp.

Treatment. This is by drainage via the gingival crevice and/or incision of the abscess, hot saline mouthwashes and, where indicated by the patient's general condition, with general antibiotics. Extraction of the tooth may be necessary in some cases and the patient will need periodontal care in the future.

Thrush

This is a fungus infection of the mucous membrane of the mouth by a yeast, *Candida albicans*. It is commonest in infants but is also found occasionally in adults. It is due to a change in the balance of the oral bacteria brought about by unclean conditions, such as unsterilized feeding bottles bottles and teats or dirty dentures, poor health or occasionally as the result of prolonged antibiotic or other therapy. It can affect all parts of the oral mucosa, but is more commonly found on the cheeks and tongue. It occurs as creamy-white patches which can be wiped off leaving a reddened area of mucosa.

Treatment. Attention must be paid to the causative factors, and fungicidal drugs such as nystatin applied to the lesions.

CHAPTER TWELVE

Anaesthesia

Anaesthesia is the loss of feeling or sensation in some part of the body due to a nervous lesion, anaesthetic agent or loss of consciousness. In surgery it is the term commonly used to denote loss of pain sensation produced in order that painful operations on the body can be performed. Anaesthetics are the drugs or chemical agents used to produce anaesthesia.

TYPES OF ANAESTHESIA

Local anaesthetics
These stop sensory nerve conduction by causing a reversible block to conduction along the nerve fibre and thus prevent sensation in a limited part of the body adjacent to the site of their injection or application, without loss of consciousness. (*Note:* some authorities prefer to use the term *analgesia* to describe this condition more precisely, for although pain sensation is eliminated some sense of pressure may remain. This descriptive precision in defining the two closely similar conditions is not yet universally used throughout the dental profession, but it is important to recognize the difference.) Topical or surface anaesthesia is a form of local anaesthesia produced by the application of a suitable agent to the surface of the skin or mucous membrane.

Regional anaesthesia
This is also called nerve block and is produced when a local anaesthetic drug is injected into the neighbourhood of a selected sensory nerve to block nerve conduction from a region of the body.

Relative analgesia
This is a method of inhalation sedation and analgesia produced by the administration of low concentrations of nitrous oxide to patients who remain conscious.

General anaesthesia
This is when drugs are given before and during surgical procedures to produce a state of unconsciousness and loss of painful sensations and also to

induce muscle relaxation. General anaesthetic agents are usually administered by allowing the patient to breathe in gases and vapours (inhalation anaesthesia) or by injection of a solution of the drug into a vein (intravenous anaesthesia).

INDICATIONS AND CHOICE

Anaesthetic drugs must not be given without careful consideration of the need for anaesthesia and the patient's condition on *every* occasion. All anaesthesia is an abnormal state produced with some degree of risk, however small, and should only be given when the relief more than compensates for the poisonous effect.

The preoperative assessment of the patient will include consideration of fitness for operation, age, weight, the general health with particular reference to the cardiovascular, respiratory and central nervous systems and finally the emotional condition and the need for preoperative sedation.

The type of anaesthetic used is dictated by the region, duration, noise and difficulty of the operation as well as the presence of infection and the patient's preference.

Choosing the type of anaesthesia

Local or regional anaesthesia. This is usually indicated for routine dental procedures frequently repeated (such as a course of conservation treatment), within limited areas and where there is no local infection that would be dispersed into the tissues by injection. It is also useful when the patient is unfit for general anaesthesia, for example, in respiratory disorders.

Topical anaesthesia. This can be used in the mouth prior to local anaesthetic injection or on its own to assist surface procedures, such as deep scaling, fitting matrix bands, to prevent 'gagging' during impression-taking and in the treatment of painful ulcers.

Relative analgesia. This is used to alleviate fear and improve patient cooperation. There is a certain extent of analgesia, but pain is further controlled by the use of local anaesthetic agents.

General anaesthesia. This is indicated for operation in more than one quadrant of the mouth at once, in the presence of infection at the operation site (such as a dental abscess) and for very young children or apprehensive or mentally handicapped patients of all ages. Many dental procedures are of short duration and can be carried out under general anaesthesia in the dental surgery; for longer operations, extensive surgery requiring endotracheal intubation, or ill-health, the patient should be admitted to hospital.

LOCAL ANAESTHESIA

Local anaesthetic agents are active within 5 minutes of administration and their effect usually lasts about an hour. The duration of action of injected local anaesthetic drugs is increased if adrenaline is added to the solution to cause local vasoconstriction. Most local anaesthetic solutions contain the agent, adrenaline (or some other vasoconstricting drug), a trace of antiseptic and saline carefully balanced to prevent irritation of the tissues. Adrenaline is contraindicated in cardiovascular disease and certain medical conditions.

Lignocaine hydrochloride (Xylocaine). This is used in a 2 per cent solution with adrenaline, producing extensive profound and prolonged anaesthesia. Lignocaine is also a very effective topical anaesthetic agent used in an ointment containing 5 per cent of the drug in a pleasantly flavoured base and in 4 percent sprays or solutions.

Prilocaine hydrochloride (Citanest). This is a local anaesthetic of low toxicity which is similar to lignocaine. It is used in a 4 per cent solution plain, or in a 3 per cent solution with felypressin as a vasoconstrictor. It may be given to patients whose medical condition contraindicates adrenaline, for example, those with heart problems or high blood pressure (hypertension). Felypressin should *not* be used for pregnant women. Excessive amounts of local anaesthetic solutions must never be given and they must be used with care in every case.

ADMINISTRATION

Topical anaesthetic agents. These are conveyed by a pledget of cottonwool or a spray to the dried mucosal surface of the mouth. Their action is complete in 2 to 5 minutes and reduced if saliva washes the drug away prematurely.

Local anaesthetic solutions. These are injected with a syringe, commonly a dental cartridge syringe (with or without an aspirating action). The dental cartridge consists of 2ml of sterile local anaesthetic solution contained in a glass tube sealed at each end and it should remain in its sealed, sterile package until it is required. The cartridge is loaded into the sterile metal syringe framework where the syringe piston comes in contact with the rubber bung in the end of the glass tube. A sterile double-ended hypodermic needle attached to the other end of the syringe perforates the cap of the sealed tube so that pressure on the piston causes the solution to be expelled through the hollow needle. Needles are supplied in gamma-ray sterilized plastic containers. Needles should be used only on one occasion to eliminate the risk of cross-infection.

Before a patient is given a local anaesthetic a check should be made to ensure that they *have* eaten recently, and if not they should be given a glucose drink, for a low blood sugar increases any tendency to faint after injection. The patient should always be reassured and everything done to allay his apprehension prior to an injection.

Infiltration

The tip of the hypodermic needle penetrates the surface mucosa and the solution is injected slowly to allow it to diffuse into the deeper tissues.

All upper permanent teeth, lower incisors and canines and all primary teeth and their associated soft tissues and bone can be anaesthetized by infiltrating the solution over the apex of the tooth on both sides of the alveolus. Smaller quantities are used for children.

Periodontal ligament injection

This method uses a special syringe capable of injecting small increments of solution under high pressure. The patient is first given an antiseptic mouthwash. Then the tip of the needle is advanced down the gingival crevice until a small amount of the solution can be injected into the periodontal membrane. The gingival condition must be healthy or infection may be carried to the injection site.

Inferior dental nerve block

This requires a long needle of larger diameter than that used for infiltration anaesthesia. Deep injections like this require that an aspirating syringe is used. This allows the operator to make sure that the tip of the needle has not penetrated a deep vessel. With the patient's mouth wide open, the needle penetrates the mucosa behind the mandibular third molar region and slightly above the occlusal plane with the barrel of the syringe over the premolar region on the opposite side of the mandible. The needle is advanced along the inner surface of the ramus of the mandible until the tip lies next to the inferior dental and lingual nerves before the solution is slowly injected. This will anaesthetize the whole area served by these two nerves, including the pulps of the premolar and molar teeth and the lingual mucosa on that side. The patient will also be aware of a loss of sensation in the lower lip on the injected side. A further infiltration injection on the buccal aspect of these teeth will act upon the long buccal nerve serving the buccal mucosa and complete the anaesthesia required for extractions in the region.

Complication

Injection of the wrong drug. Always double-check the contents of the syringe with the dental surgeon.

Injection techniques (Table 1)

Table 1 Local anaesthesia for teeth

	Teeth and associated tissues	Nerve supply	Injections used
$\underline{87}$ | $\underline{78}$	Pulps, roots and periodontal structures Alveolar bone Buccal mucoperiosteum (gum) Palatal mucoperiosteum	Posterior superior alveolar nerve Greater palatine nerve	Buccal infiltration by the tooth Palatal infiltration by the tooth
$\underline{6}$ | $\underline{6}$	Pulps, roots and periodontal structures Alveolar bone Buccal mucoperiosteum Palatal mucoperiosteum	Posterior and middle superior alveolar nerves Greater palatine nerve	Buccal infiltration by the tooth Palatal infiltration by the tooth
$\underline{54}$ | $\underline{45}$	Pulps, both roots and periodontal structures Alveolar bone Labial mucoperiosteum Palatal mucoperiosteum	Posterior and middle superior alveolar nerves Greater palatine nerve	Buccal infiltration opposite apex Palatal infiltration at level of apex
$\underline{321}$ | $\underline{123}$	Pulps, roots and periodontal structures Alveolar bone Buccal mucoperiosteum Palatal mucoperiosteum	Anterior superior alveolar nerve Labial branches of infraorbital nerve Long sphenopalatine nerve Long sphenopalatine nerve	Labial infiltration at level of apex Palatal infiltration
$\underline{8\text{-}4}$ | $\underline{4\text{-}8}$	Pulps, roots and periodontal structures Aleveolar bone Buccal mucoperiosteum Lingual mucoperiosteum	Inferior dental nerve Buccal nerve Mental nerve Lingual nerve	Inferior dental nerve block which also includes lingual nerve block Buccal infiltration by side of tooth Lingual nerve block
$\underline{3\text{-}1}$ | $\underline{1\text{-}3}$	Pulps, roots and periodontal structures Alveolar bone Labial mucoperiosteum Lingual mucoperiosteum	Incisive branch of inferior dental nerve Mental nerve Lingual nerve	Labial infiltration at the apex Lingual infiltration at the apex Jointly with labial infiltration Lingual infiltration at apex

Injection into a vessel. The general circulation of the local anaesthetic solution will make the patient's heart beat faster and make him feel unwell.

Patient faints or collapses. See section on Emergencies, page 217.

Damage to the anaesthetized parts. Always manipulate or retract anaesthetized regions with care and gentleness. Warn the patient not to eat or smoke before the anaesthetic has worn off completely, and to avoid very hot drinks.

Out-of-date drugs. Never use anaesthetic solution that has become discoloured for it may be less potent, irritant or contaminated.
Note: Hypodermic needles must be handled with care to prevent needlestick injuries. Special precautions when resheathing a used needle can include the use of bulky sheath holders (such as the Ash Jenker), which allow it to be done with only one hand.

GENERAL ANAESTHETIC AGENTS AND APPARATUS

The ideal general anaesthetic agent must be reversible, controllable, predictable, safe and have minimal side-effects. Many different drugs and techniques are used in dental surgery and the DSA should be well-rehearsed in her duties by the other members of the team before she assists with any case treated under general anaesthesia.

Inhalation anaesthesia
Nitrous oxide (dental gas). This is a colourless, non-inflammable gas supplied in metal cylinders. It is the safest general anaesthetic agent if used correctly and allows quick recovery. In use it requires a marked reduction of the patient's circulating oxygen level and can be used alone only for very brief operations. In resistant patients other stronger anaesthetic agents have to be added to nitrous oxide to allow increased oxygen to be given if an operation lasts more than 2 minutes.

Halothane (Fluothane). This is a colourless, volatile, non-inflammable liquid. It is a widely used agent, non-irritant, pleasant to inhale and with a low incidence of postoperative sickness. It is used in short procedures requiring rapid recovery, and may be combined with nitrous oxide and oxygen for dental anaesthesia. It can effect the heart rate and cause a fall in blood pressure during anaesthesia. It should not be used more than once every 4 to 6 months for a particular patient or it may cause liver function problems or jaundice. The dental team must make sure that there is adequate ventilation in the surgery when halothane is used, or they may suffer these cumulative effects themselves.

Enflurane (Ethrane). This is a volatile anaesthetic agent similar to halothane and used in the same way. It is pleasant for the patient and takes effect quickly. It has a marked cardiorespiratory depressant effect but repeated use does not seem to affect the liver.

Trichloroethylene (Trilene). This is a volatile, blue-dyed, non-inflammable liquid that can decompose to a poisonous gas if heated or if it comes into contact with strong alkalis in a closed-circuit anaesthetic apparatus. Its vapours are generally mixed with nitrous oxide and oxygen for dental anaesthesia. Disadvantages with its use are that recovery is often delayed, and postoperative vomiting occurs frequently.

Apparatus

The *inhalation anaesthetic apparatus* usually supports several *gas and oxygen cylinders* (which must be labelled 'full' or 'in use' so that they never run out without warning) whose flow passes through *pressure-reducing valves* and *flow controls* and is monitored by *flowmeters* as it passes through flexible tubing to the patient. The flow can be diverted through *vaporizing bottles* in order to take up volatile agents and a balloon-like *breathing bag* is included in the stream. The gases and vapours are delivered for the patient to inhale them via a *nose-piece or face-piece* (mask) and breathed out again through an *expiration valve* attached to it.

The *relative analgesia apparatus* is very similar but with two important differences:

1. The apparatus is preset so that it will not deliver less than 30 per cent oxygen, and has a device that cuts off the nitrous oxide flow if the oxygen runs out.
2. There is no provision for adding any other volatile agent to the mixture. The apparatus cannot produce anaesthesia.

RELATIVE ANALGESIA (RA)

See Fig. 12/1.

Low concentrations of nitrous oxide in oxygen are given by inhalation to patients who *remain conscious*. The amount of nitrous oxide administered can be controlled within fine limits to suit a particular patient's needs. The gases may be given by the operator because of the high safety factors built into the apparatus. (This is the only circumstance where an anaesthetic agent may be administered to the patient by the operator. The use of a *general anaesthetic* requires the presence of a trained anaesthetist to give single-minded constant attention to the patient's condition.)

Relative analgesia must not be given in certain circumstances, for

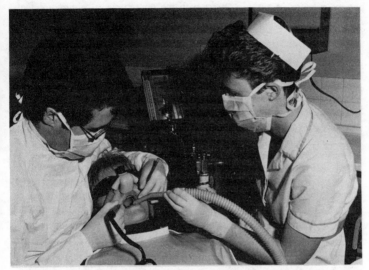

Fig. 12/1 Cavity preparation under relative analgesia. The DSA uses the high-speed suction tip to evacuate the handpiece water spray residue and saliva

example upper respiratory infections (colds, etc.), lung disease, heart disease, certain general illnesses, active psychiatric disorders, complicated medication and in pregnancy.

Relative analgesia is indicated to help overcome the patient's fear of dental treatment, excessive gagging or inability to undergo prolonged treatment sessions.

Preparation. Make sure the apparatus is turned on and that the cylinders are adequately filled; that is, if two cylinders are partially used then the other two must be full and ready for use.

Although relative analgesia may be given soon after the patient has taken a light meal, it is best to keep the food intake to a minimum.

The operation
The patient sits comfortably in the chair, a suitable-sized nose-piece is adjusted into place. The operator talks in a reassuring and encouraging manner explaining the sensations that the patient is feeling such as 'warm and tingling, floating on a magic carpet', etc., while adjusting the combined flow of nitrous oxide and oxygen both in proportions and total flow level to

suit the needs of the patient. Induction will take several calm minutes. The patient remains in verbal contact with the operator at all times but feels relaxed and happy and reacts sluggishly. He will still need local anaesthesia for painful procedures. Towards the end of the session the oxygen proportion is gradually raised to 100 per cent to ensure speedy recovery. Finally the patient should sit in the chair, breathing normal air, for 5 minutes before leaving.

STAGES OF ANAESTHESIA

As the anaesthetic agent is taken in the patient passes through a sequence of stages of anaesthesia.

Stage 1: Analgesia (progressive loss of sensation to painful stimuli).
Stage 2: Delirium (unconscious, but reacts to stimuli such as noise).
Stage 3: Unconscious (with muscular relaxation – surgical anaesthesia).
Stage 4: Respiratory paralysis (the patient can only be kept alive by artificial respiration).

The anaesthetist can judge the stage at which the patient is being maintained by attention to such things as the patient's respiration rate, the skin colour, the eyes and so on. Oxygen and stimulant drugs should be available whenever a general anaesthetic is given.

INHALATION ANAESTHESIA

Preparation of the patient
The anaesthetist will check that the apparatus is switched on and in working order. He may need assistance from the DSA with regard to changing empty gas cylinders for full ones.

The patient should have signed his consent form for being given an anaesthetic. A parent or guardian must sign for a child under 16 years. He must *not* have taken food or drink for at least 4 hours before receiving a general anaesthetic to avoid the danger of inhaling vomit while unconscious. He should visit the toilet before going into the surgery.

The patient's identity is confirmed so that the correct records and radiographs are available. After the anaesthetist has examined him, the patient is seated in the chair, his collar and any other tight clothing that might impede respiration is loosened, any dentures are removed. In most cases a restraining strap is fastened round his waist as a seat belt and he is asked to interlock the fingers of each hand before the all-enveloping bib is put over him. The dental surgeon may again ask the patient his name, and briefly examines the teeth to be extracted and places a mouth prop in position unless the anaesthetist would prefer the prop to be inserted at a later stage.

The operation

The operating light is turned off and the anaesthetist starts to administer the anaesthetic. Strict silence is observed in the room during this induction period. The DSA must be prepared with all the instruments required, but must also pay attention to the anaesthetist. When anaesthesia is achieved the DSA must switch on the operating light while the dental surgeon packs off the patient's mouth with a long gauze swab leaving the nasopharynx free for respiration. The DSA will then assist as required, this may include passing instruments, retracting and using a sucker tube. If the operation switches from one side of the mouth to the other the prop has to be changed over with the help of an expanding Mason's gag to hold the jaws open. The dental surgeon will remove the pack and the prop at the end of the operation. The anaesthetist will support the patient's head and check the airway.

Some surgeons, with the anaesthetist's permission, place a gauze socket pack in position over the extraction wounds, ensuring that a long end of the pack projects from the patient's mouth.

Postoperative care

When the operation ends the DSA will remain with the patient during the first recovery period with a kidney dish to hand for him to spit into or in case of vomiting. *At no time whatsoever during the recovery stage should the unconscious patient be left unaccompanied.* As consciousness returns a few soothing words will help the patient to reorientate himself. Unless a trolley is available the patient may have to be assisted by two people to the recovery room to lie down for a while before going home, but nothing should be done to make him feel rushed at this stage of recovery.

The surgeon must satisfy himself that all the bleeding has stopped and the patient is physically fit to be discharged, before he can be allowed to leave.

Complications

Prolonged general anaesthesia with the unconscious patient in an upright position is ill-advised, because a fall in blood pressure may result in poor circulation and oxygen deprivation to the head and the risk of brain damage.

With a totally unconscious patient under a short-acting, yet potent, anaesthetic undergoing an operation in the region of the airway extreme vigilance is required to prevent any injury or untoward reaction. He must never be left alone. His position in the chair must remain satisfactory to avoid twisting his arms; he must be protected from injury by hot instruments, etc.; his airway must be maintained clear and protected from foreign matter such as blood, vomit, pack or tooth. Where the patient leaves the surgery on a trolley and is still unconscious, he should be placed in the recovery position, on his side and the airway protected by supporting the chin well forward as directed by the anaesthetist.

Following a general anaesthetic the patient should be escorted home by a responsible adult and forbidden to drive a car or work machinery for at least the rest of that day.

INTRAVENOUS ANAESTHESIA

An intravenous anaesthetic agent can be administered as a basal anaesthetic and followed up immediately by an inhalation anaesthetic in cases of difficult induction or fear of 'the mask'. Intravenous anaesthetics may also be used safely and effectively to produce a condition just short of surgical anaesthesia that is satisfactory for extraction or conservation of teeth. All intravenous methods should only be used by experienced skilled anaesthetists with full facilities and competence to deal with respiratory or cardiac complications. These drugs must *not* be given in certain medical conditions, for example, liver disease.

Thiopentone sodium (Pentothal) is a yellow-white powder that is soluble in water. Given intravenously in a 2.5 per cent freshly made-up solution it produces rapid anaesthesia which can be prolonged by further small doses at intervals. Recovery is fairly rapid.

Other intravenous anaesthetic agents include *methohexitone sodium* (Brietal sodium) and *propofol* (Diprivan) both of which allow a more rapid recovery. *Diazepam* (Valium) and *midazolam* (Hypnoval) are sometimes used to produce sedation and amnesia (as in *intravenous sedation* for prolonged dental procedures).

Preparation of the patient

This is the same as for an inhalation anaesthetic. The patient then lies down on his back (supine) (an advantage because it maintains a good circulation to the brain at all times). One sleeve, generally the left, is rolled up to expose the arm. Gripping and compressing the arm above the elbow (by the DSA in most cases) will cause the veins on the forearm and hand to standout so that the anaesthetist can select and penetrate an appropriate vessel with the hypodermic needle. Before making an injection the skin is cleaned with an alcohol swab. As the drug is injected the compression is released. Where incremental doses are required arrangements are made to hold the needle in the vein by one of several methods and the patient's arm may be supported during the operation by strapping it to a rigid, gutter-like splint attached to the chair. The patient's eyes must be protected with gauze pads (double eye pads) while he is supine. During the operation the airway must be protected from debris, blood and other fluids by the use of absorbent packs and high-velocity suction. For in-patients in hospital this is made more certain when an endotracheal tube is passed into the trachea and the throat packed off by the anaesthetist. A laryngoscope is used to allow the anaesthetist to see and illuminate the opening of the larynx.

Some anaesthetists now use electronic monitoring devices attached to the patient to check continuously the patient's reactions to the anaesthetic, such as oxygen saturation levels, pulse rate and pulse volume.

At the end of the operation the anaesthetist will require the sucker with wide-bore nozzle to complete the protection of the airway as the pack is removed.

Postoperative care

The patient is usually moved to the recovery room on a trolley as before. During the recovery period the patient is generally asked to lie on his side and spit out into a kidney dish. He should lie still in a quiet room until recovered enough to sit up comfortably. He should then sit in a chair for a further period before leaving the surgery. Once again he should only be discharged by the dental surgeon himself. As with inhalation anaesthesia he should be escorted home by another adult and forbidden to drive or operate machinery for the rest of that day.

Postoperative instructions to the patient – such as what to do in the event of persistent bleeding or severe pain – should be given on a printed card so that they are remembered.

Complications

These are rare if cases are carefully selected for this type of anaesthesia. The unconscious patient must be protected at all times as described in the section on inhalation anaesthesia. In the unlikely event of drug overdose the patient will require supportive measures by the anaesthetist to maintain the respiration and circulation until the drug effect wears off.

Intravenous injection must be carried out with care for if any of the drug is deposited in the tissues outside the vein it may cause postoperative pain and irritation in the region.

Emergencies

1. Keep the team alert, trained and rehearsed in the treatment of emergencies and complications that may be associated with the administration of anaesthetic drugs. (See Chapter 18, Emergencies.)
2. Make sure that the *emergency kit* is always available, fully stocked and ready for use.

CHAPTER THIRTEEN

Oral Surgery

Oral surgery is the branch of surgery concerned with operations that are carried out on the jaws and associated soft tissues.

Treatment planning for surgery must be based on a thorough case history and diagnostic system with special attention to the patient's medical history and fitness for operation. Each operation should be planned carefully with step-by-step consideration of every stage including premedication (sedative or antibiotic), anaesthetic, operative technique, provisions for possible complications and postoperative care. Surgery must be carried out under strictly aseptic conditions to prevent wound cross-infection. The patient's records, including dental radiographs, must be available in the surgery for reference during any operation.

EXTRACTION OF TEETH

Extraction means the process of removing or drawing out a tooth from the mouth.

Teeth have to be extracted for many reasons including acute or chronic infection, grossly broken down teeth that cannot be conserved, impaction, supernumerary teeth, trauma and for orthodontic reasons.

Forceps

Dental forceps (Figs 13/1 and 13/2) are designed to grip erupted teeth firmly at the neck. They are composed of handles, joint and beaks. They are made in a wide variety of shapes to fit the various anatomical contours of the teeth, to allow access to teeth in different regions of the mouth and also to suit the operator's personal preference.

Forceps extraction technique

The operator holds the forceps with the little finger between the handles to open the beaks. The blades of the beaks are inserted under the gingival margin and the forceps pressed up firmly before closing the handles to grip the tooth on cementum. The grip must be firm, but care must be taken not to crush the tooth and break it.

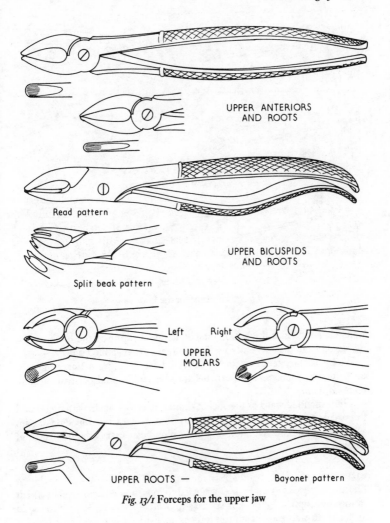

UPPER ANTERIORS
AND ROOTS

Read pattern

Split beak pattern

UPPER BICUSPIDS
AND ROOTS

Left   Right

UPPER
MOLARS

UPPER ROOTS —   Bayonet pattern

Fig. 13/1 Forceps for the upper jaw

The tooth, forceps and arm are now a single lever used to enlarge the socket containing the tooth. The tooth is moved firmly in directions that will expand the socket and these forces vary according to the anatomy of the tooth but are mainly in the direction of the thinner, weaker buccal plate. Some teeth, such as the upper central incisors, can be rotated. Finally, with the

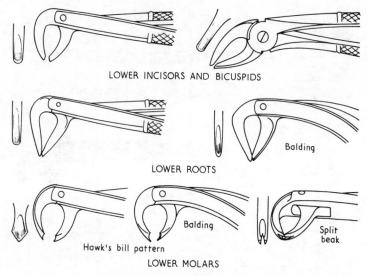

LOWER INCISORS AND BICUSPIDS

LOWER ROOTS

Balding

Hawk's bill pattern

Balding

Split beak

LOWER MOLARS

Fig. 13/2 Forceps for the lower jaw

walls expanded and the periodontal attachment ruptured the tooth can be delivered from the socket. Note that teeth are never 'pulled out'.

When primary teeth are being extracted for a child great care must be taken not to damage or disturb the forming, unerupted permanent teeth beneath them.

The expanded walls of the socket should be closed again with finger and thumb pressure to reduce the possibility of post-extraction bleeding or pain and to promote the retention of a good blood clot that is the first stage of healing.

Elevators

Elevators (Figs 13/3 and 13/4) are used to loosen and remove teeth which cannot be gripped by forceps such as impacted teeth, to remove roots, to loosen teeth before application of forceps, to divide or split teeth or to remove bone between roots.

They are made in a very wide range of shapes both in blade, shank and handle.

The further division into 'left' and 'right' indicates the inclinations of the particular blades.

An elevator may be regarded first as a *wedge*, the sharp end being forced

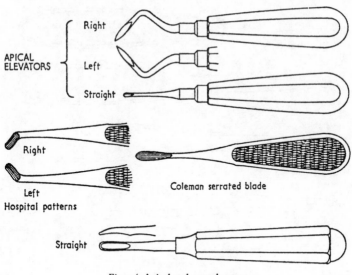

APICAL
ELEVATORS
{
Right
Left
Straight

Right

Left
Hospital patterns

Coleman serrated blade

Straight

Fig. 13/3 Apical and root elevators

between the wall of the socket and the root, and then as a *lever* to move the root. They have to be used with great care because of the powerful leverage that can be generated. In some cases their action can be greatly assisted by the use of a bur to remove bone and allow their better access to the tooth.

SURGICAL EXTRACTIONS

In certain situations, such as broken roots or impacted teeth, an incision is made so that the overlying mucoperiosteum can be reflected away in a flap from the region, and some overlying bone removed to allow better access to the tooth or root.

The flap incision is planned so that the reflected piece of mucoperiosteum is large enough to allow adequate access to the underlying tissues. The flap must have a broad base to give it a good nerve and blood supply and to encourage postoperative healing. The incision must not sever important blood vessels or nerves in the region. The incision is made with a sharp *scalpel*, the bleeding sucked away immediately to allow good visibility. The flap is next stripped back with a *periosteal elevator* to uncover the bone and may then be held away from the operation site with a suitable *retractor*, for example, the Austin retractor. Larger retractors may also be used to retract cheek, tongue, and so on.

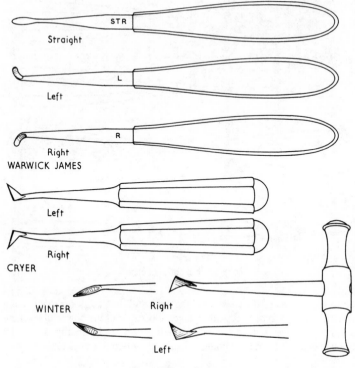

Fig. 13/4 Root elevators

Bone may be removed with suitable *surgical burs* or, under general anaesthesia, *chisels* and a *mallet* to allow access to the underlying tooth (Fig. 13/5). After the extraction is completed the margins of the bony wound may require smoothing with bone nibbling forceps or *rongeurs* and *files* before the wound is irrigated with sterile saline and closed. The flap is repositioned and sutured into place.

The sutures used intraorally are generally of black braided silk. Occasionally resorbable catgut may be used because it does not have to be removed subsequently. Half-circle cutting edge needles are used in the mouth and ready-threaded eyeless needles are obtainable in sterile packs.

The margin of the flap is gripped with toothed forceps, the curved needle is held in a pair of artery forceps (Spencer-Wells) or one of a range of special needle-holders. The needle is passed through the tissues, on either side of the incision line, the thread drawn after it and then knotted into place. Single

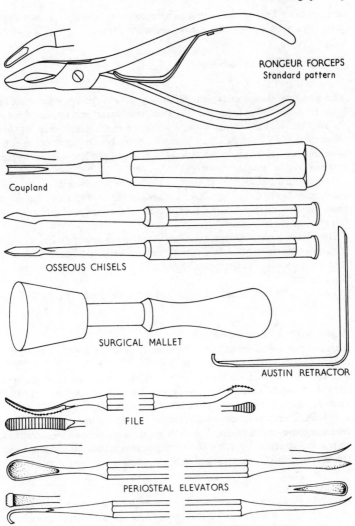

RONGEUR FORCEPS
Standard pattern

Coupland

OSSEOUS CHISELS

SURGICAL MALLET

AUSTIN RETRACTOR

FILE

PERIOSTEAL ELEVATORS

Fig. 13/5 Bone operating instruments

or interrupted sutures are commonly used and after each knot the excess suture thread is cut away by the assistant with sharp scissors before the next suture is placed.

Sutures hold the tissues together, prevent haemorrhage, reduce infection and promote healing. Silk sutures have to be removed in 4 to 7 days, generally a simple procedure not requiring anaesthesia.

SPECIAL OPERATIONS

Impacted teeth

Those teeth whose normal eruptions into the mouth is prevented by adjacent teeth are described as impacted. The teeth most commonly squeezed out of the arch are third molars and canines which are much later in erupting than others alongside. Impacted teeth may sometimes be symptomless but more commonly give rise to pain (which may be referred to other parts of the face and head) or to local infections.

Lower third molars may lie impacted in a variety of inclinations; mesio-angular, distoangular, vertical and horizontal and also at a variable depth from the occlusal plane. They thus present a wide range of difficulty and require expert assessment.

Broadly, the tooth is approached via a mucoperiosteal flap and with the removal of overlying bone. In some cases a large tooth is deliberately divided with a bur or chisel, to allow it to be delivered through a small exit in two or three pieces.

Canine teeth may often be approached surgically from the palatal side of the arch.

Apicectomy (root amputation)

This is a method of dealing with infected tissue at the apex of a tooth that cannot be resolved by root canal therapy.

The tooth may be root-filled prior to operation or in some cases the open apex of the tooth is sealed with amalgam at the time of operation. A flap is made to expose bone over the affected apex and the overlying bone removed with burs. The apex is defined and cut off leaving at least two-thirds of the remaining root undisturbed. The diseased tissue is scraped away, *curetted*, with a spoon-shaped curette, the bone margins smoothed, irrigated with sterile saline and the flap sutured back into place.

Simple cysts

Again the overlying mucoperiosteal flap is retracted and bone is removed to expose the cyst lining. Small cysts can be curetted away entirely, *enucleated*, and the cavity closed with the flap to heal normally. Large bone cysts may have to be allowed to collapse over a period by *marsupializing* them. The superficial wall of the cyst is cut away and the opening made to persist by inserting a suitable plug. Each day the pouch of the cyst cavity is washed clean and the plug replaced. Rapidly, over the course of weeks, quite large cyst cavities will collapse and fill up from the bottom with new bone.

Prosthetic preparation

A wide range of operations may be carried out to facilitate the construction of dentures. Bone and soft tissue contours of the ridges, bony swellings on the hard palate, and the depths of sulci can all be changed surgically. Where multiple extractions have been carried out, removal of interradicular bony septa (the segments of bone and socket wall between the teeth) and collapse of the labial walls of the sockets can overcome maxillary protrusion, for example.

Dental implants. These are used occasionally and there are many techniques. For example, in two consecutive operations (the first for bone preparation and an impression) a prepared metal framework is placed in contact with the shaped bone of the ridge and the mucosa sewn back into place, leaving locating studs projecting through the tissues into the mouth. The denture superstructure is made to fit on these studs and gains considerable retention in this way (see p.178).

Biopsy

The tissue to be examined is removed using a scalpel and toothed dissecting forceps and transferred to a screw-capped specimen bottle containing preservative solution such as 10 per cent formolsaline. The bottle must be clearly labelled and accompanied by a short history of the condition and instructions, when despatched to the laboratory. (Check with the pathology laboratory of the local hospital about special precautions to be taken if the specimens are to be sent to them by post.)

Abscess drainage

Occasionally an abscess is neglected or occurs so quickly that by the time the patient arrives at the dental surgery a considerable swelling has occurred. When necessary, in addition to antibiotic therapy and extraction or opening a tooth to drain via the root canal, the soft tissue swelling has to be incised to let out the accumulated pus.

Intraoral incisions may be made into the centre of the abscess (where it 'points') with a scalpel. Though rarely necessary, extraoral drainage is also carried out by incision, taking great care not to sever arteries or nerves and may be further assisted by blunt dissection with artery forceps. Extraoral wounds should be covered with a dry dressing.

Dislocated mandible

The jaw may become fixed in the open position by a blow or an extraction of a lower tooth in a patient with lax joint ligaments. The condition is overcome by the operator pressing the mandible downwards and backwards with his protected thumbs on the posterior teeth. The condition should be corrected as soon as possible and a general anaesthetic may be required.

Oroantral fistula

This is an opening between the mouth and the maxillary antrum and can occur following the extraction of a tooth whose roots were closely associated with the floor of the antrum. Small openings usually seal with blood clot and heal uneventfully. Large openings should be repaired immediately with a buccal flap. An established fistula links the two cavities with an epithelial-lined channel and the patient suffers the effects of an inflamed antral lining, etc.

POSTOPERATIVE CARE

Haemorrhage

The patient should not be allowed to leave the surgery until all bleeding has ceased. He should be given careful instructions not to disturb the clot, not to use excessive mouthwashes or take very hot food or drinks and to avoid alcohol and excessive bodily activity for the next 24 hours. He should be advised how to aply haemostatic pressure to the wound by biting on a firm pad, such as a clean handkerchief, should bleeding recur (see Chapter 18).

Pain

The patient should be given a supply of a mild analgesic drug such as aspirin or paracetamol for use should postoperative pain occur.

Infection

An aseptic technique should minimize this complication, but preoperative and postoperative antibiotic therapy may be necessary in some cases. Healing may be promoted by the use of frequent hot saline mouthwashes after the first 24 hours.

Dry socket

A localized infection of alveolar bone (osteitis) following tooth extraction. This painful condition arises due to premature loss of blood clot, perhaps due to excessive mouth rinsing immediately after extraction. It is more common in the mandible. Treatment involves gentle irrigation of the socket with warm saline solution and dressing it with zinc oxide/eugenol or a proprietary paste. The patient may also require antibiotics and analgesia.

Medication and anaesthetics

The patient should be made aware of the after-effects that any drugs and anaesthetic agents used may produce. Premedication usually causes drowsiness, so the patient must be accompanied by a responsible adult, as must a patient who is to have a general anaesthetic. The patient must *never* be allowed to drive a car while under the influence of these drugs.

Anxiety
The patient must be told whom to contact in an emergency should he become anxious about any postoperative aspect of the surgical treatment.

FRACTURES

Fractures of the jaws and the facial bones fall within the scope of oral surgery, but as a specialized field generally only dealt with in hospital. Many forms of fracture occur and each demands different details of treatment.

Broadly, fractured bones have to be replaced into their correct position, *reducing* the fracture, held firmly in place, *immobilization*, for the required number of weeks, the patient's general health maintained, and swelling, infection and pain combated while healing takes place. After healing, the immobilization or *fixation* is removed and the part *rehabilitated*.

Often the fractured segments of the jaws hold firm teeth and these can be fastened together and to the opposing teeth by wires or cast silver splints to immobilize the fracture. Where the angle of the fracture is not favourable for this form of immobilization or no teeth exist on the fragments, the bones may be wired together directly and the fixation achieved by pins driven into the bone extraorally and linked to each other by special screw brackets and bars perhaps extending to a firm anchorage in a plaster head cap or metal halo.

Great attention has to be paid to making up an interesting and nourishing semiliquid diet for a patient whose jaws are immobilized.

WIDER APPLICATIONS OF ORAL SURGERY

The scope of oral surgery extends into and links up with the fields of general surgery (in the treatment of tumours, extensive head and neck injuries), plastic surgery, and many dental techniques are of value in other fields, for example maxillofacial prostheses.

CHAPTER FOURTEEN

Prosthetic Dentistry

Prosthetic dentistry or prosthodontics is that part of restorative dentistry concerned with the construction of removable appliances to replace lost teeth. These prosthetic appliances are called dentures. They are generally described by their extent, for example, full dentures and partial dentures, and by the materials from which they are made, such as acrylic, gold, chrome-cobalt.

Although these appliances are made with extreme care, skill and ingenuity, they can never be as satisfactory as sound natural teeth.

AIMS OF DENTURE CONSTRUCTION

1. To retain masticatory function.
2. To restore and maintain good appearance and prevent changes in facial contours and temporomandibular joint function due to reduced muscular activity or loss of bite height.
3. To maintain clear speech. The loss of teeth, particularly at the front of the mouth, can hamper the pronunciation of certain sounds.
4. To prevent overeruption of unopposed teeth, tilting of teeth adjacent to a space and the production of excessive strain on the periodontal structure of the remaining teeth.

A great many different techniques are used in making dentures, but only two basic methods can be described here as common examples.

CONSTRUCTION OF COMPLETE DENTURES

Following the extraction of teeth, the sockets in the alveolus heal first by organization of the blood clot into fibrous tissue and then by conversion of this to bone. The healed alveolar bone and its overlying tissues form a ridge. This ridge will be large and broad to begin with, but gradually over the years it will resorb and reduce in size. In extreme age, or in cases where there has been extensive bone destruction due to periodontal disease before the extractions, the ridge can become very thin and shallow and present little for a denture to be based upon.

Preliminary treatment plan
A careful case history and a complete survey of the endentulous (toothless) mouth is essential plus the study of any available pre-extraction records (models or photographs) or previous dentures.

First appointment. First impressions are taken of the upper ridge and hard palate and the lower ridge using impression compound or alginate in selected stock impression trays. The laboratory instructions should indicate which type of impression material will be used for the second working impressions.

Laboratory work. The first impressions are cast by vibrating a creamy mix of plaster of Paris into them. When this has set hard the trays and impression material are removed and any surplus plaster trimmed away neatly. These models are examined and the outlines of the denture-bearing areas are marked out in pencil. Special trays, made of plastic (acrylic) are constructed on these models with their margins contoured to include the denture-bearing areas.

Second appointment. The second more accurate working impressions are taken. The special trays are tried in the mouth and adjusted as necessary to avoid muscle attachments or overextension of the margins, with files, large burs and sandpaper. Additions to the tray margins may be made with a tracing stick compound if necessary before the impressions are taken in plaster, zinc-oxide/eugenol impression paste or alginate. (Alginate impressions must not be allowed to dry out on their way to the laboratory.)

Laboratory work. The working impressions are cast in hard stone. The trays and impression materials are removed and the models trimmed. Wax *occlusion rims* are constructed on firm *base plates* of acrylic or heated moulded shellac material made to fit the denture-bearing areas.

Third appointment. The jaw relations are registered. The occlusion bite rims are tried in the mouth and the bases adjusted, if necessary, until they are a comfortable fit. The wax rims are then trimmed and contoured with a heated wax knife to indicate the amount of bulk required to support the upper lip, the occlusal plane and to register the correct amount of space between the jaws. The vertical relationship may be checked with a bite gauge or callipers to measure distances between the nose and chin both with the rims together and with the jaws in a relaxed position and the mouth empty. (These

measurements are made according to certain conventions that will differentiate between the resting position and the functional position and require
very careful judgement.) The rims are finally sealed together in the mouth
with jaw registration paste in the retruded or 'central' jaw relationship, so
that they may be reassembled in the correct position outside the mouth. The
centre line, the resting lip line, the high lip line and the corners of the mouth
are marked on the wax with the rims in position in the mouth. The make,
colour, size and shape of the teeth to be used are considered and indicated on
the laboratory instructions. (Among prosthetics specialists the old term
'taking the bite' is being superseded by the more precise term 'registering the
centric jaw relationship' and 'bite blocks' are now called 'occlusion rims'.)

Laboratory work. The models are set on a mechanical reproduction of the
jaw movement called an *articulator* in the position indicated by the bite.
Individual acrylic teeth are set up in pink wax mounted on base plates
adapted to fit these models. Great care is taken to arrange the teeth to give a
good appearance and the occlusion is checked in centric and functional
positions by movement of the articulator mechanism. Finally the waxed-up
model dentures are smoothed and contoured to the shape of the finished
appliances.

Fourth appointment. The wax model dentures are tried in the mouth. They are
cooled first in cold water so that they will not be distorted by the body heat. In
the mouth they are checked for facial and lip appearance, for occlusion in
centric and functional positions, for bite height and for size, length,
arrangement and colour of the teeth. If all is well the patient is asked to check
them visually in a hand mirror. Small adjustments of individual teeth can be
made at the chairside, out of the mouth, by warming the wax with a hot wax
knife and moving the tooth as required. More extensive alterations may mean
that the work must be returned to the laboratory and a further re-try
appointment made. When all is satisfactory, the final outlines of the dentures
are drawn on the models in pencil, with special attention to all muscle
attachments and the posterior palatal margin of the upper denture.

Laboratory work. The denture area is marked on the model with a pin-line
scratched along the pencil line indications and the posterior palatal margin of
the upper denture is cut widely into the model so that a ridge will be formed
on the denture (the post-dam seal). The wax dentures are sealed on to the
stone models at their margins and the models, plus the wax and teeth are set
into a sectional plaster mould constructed in a metal box (a dental flask) by
pouring carefully separated sections of plaster over them. When the final mix
of plaster has set, the flask is warmed in hot water until the wax softens and

then the sections of the flask can be separated so that one holds the artificial teeth firmly, the other the stone model while the walls record the contours of the rest of the denture shape. The wax can now be washed away with hot water. The cooled plaster is coated with a sodium alginate separating paint ('cold mould seal') carefully avoiding the teeth and then a fresh mix of soft acrylic dough is packed into the mould. The flask is reassembled and placed under pressure until all the excess acrylic is extruded and the flask closed firmly. The closed flask is clamped and heated in a water bath as necessary. When the acrylic has been processed (cured) and hardened the flask is cooled and then opened and the denture separated from the plaster mould. The surplus material at the edges of the denture is cut away as indicated by the original pin-lines and the cut surfaces smoothed with files, burs, stones and sandpaper. The dentures are finished and polished against revolving brushes, mops and felt wheels on a large lathe first using pumice and water followed by finer polishing agents such as whiting and water until the final high polish is achieved. The fitting surface is not polished.

Fifth appointment. The finished dentures are fitted. The upper denture is inserted first and checked for border extension, appearance and retention. Retention is achieved partly by border seal and partly by the close contact between the saliva-moistened fitting surfaces of the denture and the mucosa of the palate and ridge (in the same way that two flat glass slabs hold firmly together when their contacting surfaces are wet). This intimate contact may only develop properly when the denture has been worn for a few days. Next the lower denture is inserted and examined. The retention of the lower denture depends mainly on muscular control with the lips, cheeks and tongue and the elimination of any displacing forces as well as the wet contact of the fitting surface and mucosa. The occlusion is checked in centric and functional positions. If necessary a small amount of a gum denture fixative may be used to hold the dentures firmly and increase the patient's confidence. The patient now checks the appearance again in a hand mirror. The patient is shown how to remove and insert the dentures, told how to clean them and usually advised about how long to wear them each day. He is also recommended to eat carefully until the dentures are fully settled in and adjusted. They must certainly be worn for several hours immediately preceding the next follow-up appointment.

Sixth appointment. The patient returns after an interval of a few days for a check-up to allow the dental surgeon to hear and see how he is progressing with the dentures. The denture-bearing areas are examined for signs of inflammation or ulcers caused by excessive pressure points and the dentures eased and adjusted as necessary. The occlusion is also checked and adjusted.

When all is well, the patient is asked to return if necessary for further small adjustments, but in any case to return in 1 year for reassessment. All full dentures need check-ups and adjustments at intervals and it is unwise to neglect them indefinitely.

CONSTRUCTION OF PARTIAL DENTURES

Partial dentures are constructed to replace a missing tooth or group of teeth in a functional and aesthetic way. They take their support partly from the mucosa and partly from the remaining natural teeth by means of *clasps* (supporting arms attached to the denture and in contact with a natural tooth) and *occlusal rests* (rigid extensions lapping over the occlusal surfaces to resist occlusal pressure that could drive the denture hard against the underlying mucosa). Great care must be taken in their design and construction to avoid disrupting the natural occlusion, overstressing the remaining teeth or causing damage to the oral mucosa and gingival margins.

Preliminary treatment plan. A case history and complete oral survey including radiographs of the remaining teeth are essential before deciding to construct a denture. Any necessary conservation and periodontal treatment must be completed before the working impressions are taken.

First appointment. First impressions of the upper and lower jaws are taken in selected stock trays using alginate, and a wax leaf occlusion registration made where possible (Fig. 14/1). The laboratory work-slip should indicate which material will be used for the second impression.

Laboratory work. The models are cast in plaster and special trays are constructed in plastic. (However if the dental surgeon has decided that stock tray impressions are adequate to finish the denture on, the models are cast in stone, occlusion rims are made on firm base plates and the case proceeds to 'third appointment'.)

Whenever possible the models are mounted on an articulator before the final design is made. The model is examined and *surveyed*, a technique used to choose the best path of insertion, so that clasps can be put in the most effective positions around the teeth and any undercuts (the spaces beneath overhanging teeth or tissues when looked at from the chosen line of insertion) blocked out. Occlusal rests (metal tags fashioned to lap over the occlusal surface of teeth to support the denture) and clasps are planned so that when they are seated on the teeth they will not interfere with the occlusion in centric or functional positions.

Second appointment. The final design for the finished denture should be agreed at this stage in order that any adjustments to the natural teeth may be

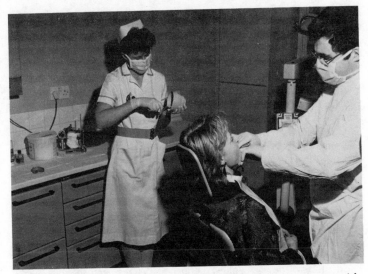

Fig. 14/1 Taking an impression. The DSA is mixing alginate impression material

made by grinding before the second impressions are taken. Finally, the accurate working impressions are taken in the special trays using an elastic impression material such as alginate.

Laboratory work. The working models are cast in hard stone and wax occlusion blocks made on firm base plates. *Note:* Some partial denture cases have so few natural teeth missing that the models can be articulated without requiring an occlusion block, although most dental technicians would prefer to have a wax leaf occlusion registration even in such a case.

Third appointment. The occlusion is registered in the mouth by trimming and marking the occlusion blocks as necessary with a wax knife. The shade of the teeth is matched with a shade guide and this is sometimes very difficult for natural teeth are rarely all the same colour in one mouth as they vary in thickness, fillings, vitality, staining, and so on.

Laboratory work. If a metal base or framework is to be used in the final denture it is now constructed in metal, for example, chrome-cobalt casting. The metal clasps and rests are contoured and fitted to the teeth (in some cases the technician prefers to leave these small structures to be made in the finishing stage). Finally the whole structure is waxed up on a base that is removable from the model – artificial teeth, clasps, rests, skeleton – and prepared for a try-in.

Fourth appointment. The model denture is tried in the mouth and checked for design, occlusion and appearance and any small adjustments made. The patient also checks the appearance in a hand mirror. Large adjustments must be made in the laboratory and checked once more at a re-try appointment before proceeding to a finish.

Laboratory work. The denture is flasked, packed, processed and finished in a similar way to a full denture.

Fifth appointment. The denture is fitted, checked again for the design, occlusion, function and appearance and any small adjustments made at the chairside. The patient is shown how to remove and replace the denture, how to clean it and the natural teeth it comes in contact with, paying particular attention to the clasped teeth.

Sixth appointment. After a few days the denture is checked again at a follow-up appointment. Any occlusal high spots or points of excessive pressure on the mucosa are eased and any other small adjustments are made. When all is well the patient is asked to return if necessary for further small adjustments. The denture will be re-examined routinely at each regular 6-monthly check-up in the future.

Cleaning dentures

The patient should be instructed to clean the dentures daily by scrubbing them with soap and water or proprietary cleanser but to be careful not to scratch the surfaces. The denture may also be soaked in a non-bleaching cleaner to remove stains, plaque and calculus.

Repairs

If a denture breaks, commonly as a result of having been mishandled out of the mouth, the technician can usually join the pieces together and effect a repair. This is fairly simple in the case of a clean fracture of acrylic when the fragments can be accurately repositioned. When there is any doubt about the positions of the pieces, or if a fragment or tooth is lost, a new impression will be required and sometimes an occlusion record of the opposing teeth. When metal has broken, the problem is more complex because it may mean removing the acrylic and teeth from a skeleton denture so that the fracture may be repaired by soldering. Close liaison with the technician is necessary to confirm the kind of impression and occlusal records he will require for a particular case.

Relines

Complete dentures will gradually loosen because of ridge resorption after they have been worn for a few years, although remaining otherwise satisfactory. New fitting surfaces may be processed into them by a relining technique.

The denture is prepared for relining by trimming flanges and any undercuts and slightly roughening the fitting surface. A zinc oxide impression paste is applied thinly to the fitting surface and the denture carefully positioned in the mouth. The opposing denture is put in the mouth and the patient instructed to close firmly so that the impression is held accurately in position and the vertical jaw relationship is not 'raised'. The peripheral margins are contoured by protuding and retracting the lips. When the paste has set, the denture and the impression it contains is sent to the laboratory. The technician casts a model and plaster overbite, cuts away the whole of the old fitting surface and processes a new one in its place. When finished and polished the result is a well-fitting appliance with the same appearance and occlusion as before.

SPECIAL APPLIANCES

Immediate dentures

These are made on models of the mouth made before the teeth are extracted. The teeth to be lost are cut away from the model during the final stages of making the denture and their acrylic replacements waxed into place. At the time of extractions, the empty sockets are immediately covered with the new denture so that the patient is at no time left without teeth. Normal healing takes place under the denture. This method is used commonly to replace anterior teeth, particularly for people who have to appear before the public or who would be embarrassed to be without teeth until healing had taken place. Immediate dentures usually require relining after about 6 months because of the post-extraction ridge shrinkage that normally occurs during this period.

Copy dentures

Copy dentures can be made to duplicate existing dentures, found to be of satisfactory construction yet loose fit, in order that a new well-fitting set can be provided. This technique can be of particular help with the aged who have come to depend upon the shape of an old denture.

Overlays

In certain circumstances, such as temporomandibular joint disturbances, overlays are constructed that cover all the occlusal surfaces of the teeth in one jaw to raise the jaw relationship to a new functional level.

Obturators

When a patient has a defective palate due to congenital cleft palate, or as a result of surgery or an accident, an obturator ('stopper') based on a denture can be constructed to seal the defect, assist speech and prevent food and liquids from leaking from the mouth to the nose. Care must be taken during the impression stage to prevent the material from passing up into the nose and perhaps getting impacted there.

Maxillofacial prostheses

Where a patient has suffered a loss of parts of the jaws, lips, nose or other parts of the face as a result of disease, injury or surgery and it is not possible to restore the parts by plastic surgery, the specialist dental team may be called in to use dental techniques and materials to make an artificial restoration of the lost tissue. These appliances can be made to look very realistic even at close quarters. This is difficult but rewarding work because successful results will allow such patients to return to normal lives in the community.

Dental implants

These are totally or partially buried structures made to help the function of inadequate dental structures. Their use is a particularly specialized field in dentistry and the subject of ongoing research. There are many classes of implants and they may be intraosseus (into bone) or extraosseus (not into bone but under the periosteum). For diadontic or endodontic implants pins are passed into the bone via the root canal of existing teeth to make them firmer (see p.167).

IMPRESSION MATERIALS

Impression materials are either rigid or elastic in character and may be thermoplastic or non-reversible.

Thermoplastic materials

Impression compound. A material made up of waxes, gums, resins and inert mineral fillers which is reversibly soft and plastic when heated and hard and rigid upon cooling. Pieces of the composition are placed in a water bath at 55 to 60°C until softened. A quantity is worked and moulded into a soft ball with the fingers, transferred to a dry metal impression tray and moulded to fit it. Any excess material is pulled off at the edge of the tray. The surface of the composition is warmed briefly over a clean flame to soften and smooth the surface and the tray and its contents are then dipped into the hot water to temper the material and ensure that no part remains flame-heated enough to burn the patient's mouth. The tray and composition is seated in place in the mouth and the cheeks, lips and tongue moved to mould the margins accurately. The impression is supported in position until the composition is cooled sufficiently to remove it from the mouth without distorting it.

Tracing stick is a composition that is softer at lower temperatures than ordinary impression composition and in pencil-thick rods may be flame-heated and used to make corrective or tissue-compressing additions to larger previous composition impressions or special trays.

Non-reversible materials

Plaster of Paris. This is dehydrated calcium sulphate and is a white, odourless and tasteless powder which can take up moisture from the air. When mixed to a smooth paste with water it sets in about 3 minutes and hardens in 15 to 20 minutes. It can be used as a rigid impression material, as well as for the construction of models and as an ingredient of investment material in casting metals. For impressions it is mixed with an anti-expansion solution, which also accelerates the setting time, containing measured amounts of salts such as potassium sulphate and borax.

A quantity of anti-expansion solution is placed in a clean rubber bowl, fine plaster of Paris powder is sprinkled evenly over the surface and allowed to soak in until a fine dry layer lies on the top. After 20 seconds the mixture is carefully spatulated, to avoid air bubbles, for 30 to 40 seconds and vibrated by banging the bowl down once or twice to cause any air bubbles that might have been produced to rise and be eliminated from the mix. The special impression tray is then filled with the mix and inserted into the mouth as the plaster starts to thicken. The setting time, usually $1\frac{1}{2}$ to 2 minutes in the mouth, is judged by observing the condition of the plaster remaining in the bowl. If the plaster breaks on removing the impression from the mouth, the fractures are clean and sharp and the pieces are easily reassembled before the impression is cast. A separating medium such as soap solution must be applied to the surface of the impression before casting it or the plaster will unite with the model material.

Commercially available impression plasters include the anti-expansion salts with the plaster in the container, and need only be mixed with water.

Impression paste. This material is rigid in character and cannot reproduce extensive undercuts. It may be used as a relining impression material and also in special trays to give an accurate working impression for an edentulous case.

Two pastes are provided, one containing, for example, oil of cloves and a resin and the other zinc oxide powder, lanolin and water. Equal quantities of the two pastes are measured out by length on a disposable mixing paper, mixing pad or a thin card and thoroughly spatulated to a creamy homogeneous consistency. White petroleum jelly is smeared on the patient's lips to prevent the paste from sticking to the skin. The paste is spread evenly over the impression surface of the tray or denture and inserted into the mouth. After about 4 to 5 minutes, when the material has hardened, the impression is removed from the mouth and inspected. Small deficiencies or air blows in the impression can be corrected by adding further small amounts of freshly mixed paste and replacing the impression in the mouth for a further period.

Alginates. These elastic, jelly-like materials, which contain some 20 per cent of inert filler, are non-reversible and can be used to reproduce undercut areas of teeth and ridge in the mouth. The gel is formed as a result of chemical action by combining a calcium salt with a solution of sodium or potassium alginate. The calcium gradually replaces the sodium and calcium alginate is precipitated in the form of an insoluble gel. When set these materials are not adhesive and must be held in the tray either mechanically, by allowing them to ooze through perforations in the tray, or by painting a sticky material on to the tray surface before loading it.

Carefully measured quantities of alginate powder and water must be used and the water must be at the correct temperature (20°C or in accordance with the manufacturer's instructions). The water is put into a rubber bowl, the powder added all at once and the materials mixed and spatulated thoroughly for some 30 seconds. The mix is loaded into the prepared tray, taking care not to overload it, and the tray positioned in the mouth. The material is allowed to set undisturbed for about 3 minutes. After removal from the mouth the material must not be allowed to dry out or the impression will become distorted. To prevent this the tray and its impression may be stored in a sealed container, such as a plastic bag, although it is better if these impressions are cast up immediately.

Note: It is dangerous to inhale alginate impression powder dust for it can give rise to lung infections. Keep the powder under control.

Synthetic rubber. See the section on indirect inlay impression technique for details of the use and mixing of this elastic, non-reversible material (p.122).

Tissue conditioners. These are plasticized acrylic materials that can be used to cover the entire fitting surface of the denture like a reline impression to produce a soft liner. They can help the tissues to recover from trauma or infection and after extractions. They also assist elderly patients who find it hard to tolerate new dentures.

DENTURE BASE MATERIAL

Acrylic resin (*methyl methacrylate*)
This popular thermoplastic denture base material is formed by the linking together of chemical molecules into chains (polymerization) to form a solid material composed of microscopic tangled masses of threads. When heated the formed material may be softened, to harden again on cooling, but it is

simpler to pack a mould with newly prepared material in dough form and allow it to polymerize to the new shape.

Acrylic resin denture base materials are supplied as a stable polymerized powder (polymer) and an unpolymerized volatile liquid (monomer). Plasticizing agents and colouring materials have been added to these constituents to improve the workability and produce the required colour.

The powder and the liquid are mixed in the recommended proportions in a glass or pottery jar and, in a short time as the reaction begins, the monomer is itself converted to polymer and links the granules of the powder together. The damp sand-like mix becomes sticky and stringy and soon forms a plastic dough. This dough is rapidly packed into the prepared flask before it becomes rubbery and the flask is closed under pressure. The clamped flask and its contents are heated in boiling water to 'cure' the material for the recommended period until the conversion of the remaining free monomer to stable polymer has been completed and the denture can proceed to the next stage.

'Cold-cure' acrylic materials are available that also contain accelerating agents and these will set completely with minimal pressure and without the application of heat. They must be used with care or free monomer may persist in the material and act as an irritant to the oral mucosa.

All acrylic resins absorb water and contract if they are allowed to dry out. Thus acrylic dentures should be stored in cold water before the patient receives them and should be kept in water when they are not in use.

Acrylic is not very resistant to abrasives and dentures should only be cleaned by brushing with soap and water and by soaking stains off with a proprietary denture bath solution if they are to retain their high polish.

CHAPTER FIFTEEN

Dentistry for Children

Paedodontics or children's dentistry includes all aspects of child dental health up to the arbitrary age of 13 years. It is mainly concerned with preventive dentistry, operative dentistry and orthodontics for this age-group and successful treatment procedures require some knowledge of basic child psychology.

The importance of child dental health cannot be overemphasized, for the first steps in dental care and in planning and carrying out any necessary dental treatment will affect the child's dental condition and attitude to treatment for the rest of its life. Every other aspect of dentistry in later years can only be in a 'follow-up' capacity. Although this chapter is devoted to child management and operative treatment for children, remember that preventive dentistry is of *prime importance* at this age.

CHILD MANAGEMENT

A child's first attitude to dentistry will be copied from the parents and other members of the family who may themselves be apprehensive about dental treatment. Some parents are ignorant of the value of the primary teeth and regard them as trivial nuisances that should be extracted if they cause trouble. Sometimes reluctance to seek treatment means that a child's mouth is neglected until severe pain or infection occurs and the child's first introduction to dentistry is unavoidably unpleasant for him.

Importance of primary teeth
Parents must be made aware of the importance of maintaining the primary teeth in a healthy condition because:

1. They are necesssary for proper mastication of a balanced diet during the child's important growing years.
2. They are part of the apparatus of speech and needed especially when the child is learning to speak.
3. They are required in the mouth to maintain space in the arch during growth of the jaws. Premature loss could aggravate possible crowding of

the permanent teeth and perhaps lead to the necessity for prolonged orthodontic treatment later.

4. The teeth play an important part in the child's appearance and their early loss may be bad for any child's self-confidence.
5. The extraction of teeth, no matter how skilfully carried out, is not a pleasant experience for a child, even if he is old enough to understand why it has to be done.

As they grow older children pass through a series of attitude changes, and it is helpful to be aware of them when the child is brought into the dental surgery.

Infant

A child's mouth plays a very important role in his general psychological make-up. At first a baby's mouth becomes a source of comfort and pleasure as he takes in milk and food to satisfy hunger pains and he gradually becomes aware of the different textures, temperatures and tastes. This connection between stomach, mouth, comfort and security becomes interwoven with many other basic themes but it always remains as a strong instinct in the subconscious. Any oral pain, discomfort or loss of teeth must therefore have a deep psychological effect as well as that at the superficial physical level, especially in the young child who cannot understand why it has happened to him.

Preschool child

Very young children often have regular sleeping periods during the afternoon and appointments should be made to avoid these times. Up to about $2\frac{1}{2}$ years old the child is strongly dependent upon his mother or mother substitute and looks to her for signals about how to react to his surroundings. He will be more upset by being separated from her than by any treatment procedure and may react best sitting or even lying on her lap. From this age any repetitive sequence of events can be used to accustom him gradually to treatment because it makes the whole thing into a game. The 'TSD' technique is useful: *Tell* the child what is to be done, 'I'm going to brush your teeth,' *Show* him the brush, 'This is the brush I'm going to brush your teeth with,' and *Do* brush his teeth, 'I'm brushing your teeth like this.'

At about $2\frac{1}{2}$ years old, most children discover that they have a personality of their own which they assert by refusing to comply with simple direct commands. It is useless to ask for their direct cooperation, but various subterfuges can help in which the child is given an apparent choice of action, for example, which of two burs should be used on his tooth, or whether he would like a warm or cold mouthwash. From this age children are very susceptible to praise about their dress or some other external feature.

At 3 years old the child wants to help and be involved in every activity. Now he understands a larger range of words and can be controlled more easily with interesting conversation. However, never let a young child discover too much about the workings of the fascinating dental equipment or he will use it as a delaying tactic and waste potential treatment time.

At 4 years old the child's self-confidence has usually expanded. He is very definite and vocal in his opinions and physically more active but is able to cooperate more readily and for longer periods. He responds to praise and being treated as a 'grown-up'. He is full of questions and these have to be answered during the continuation of treatment procedures or they become a delaying weapon. At this age a child will boast about his dental experiences later on, so make sure that his imagination has nothing unexplained to work on.

School child

At about 5 years old most children start school and this has the effect of suddenly expanding his social experience. He leaves the home environment for much of the day to become one of a large group and has to conform to new behaviour patterns, timetables and rivalries. He gets tired at the end of the day and should have morning appointments. He is more composed and able to accept prolonged dental procedures more easily. He becomes increasingly mouth conscious at this time for he is starting to shed the first of the primary teeth.

From 6 to 10 years the child progresses through a body-conscious stage in which he is more afraid of potential damage to his body than of separation from his parent. The dental drill, the injection needle, extractions, blood, and so on, are all particularly worrying at this age and their unavoidable presence has to be reduced to a minimum by careful technique and explanation.

Adolescence

Between 11 and 13 children are going through the first stages of adolescence with its general unsettling effects on self-confidence and the ability to come to terms with changes in bodily function and mental attitudes. The physical appearance becomes of marked importance in most cases and treatment of the upper incisor teeth will carry great significance from now on. Young teenage boys who have previously been regular attenders go through a stage of regarding routine dental treatment as an unnecessary convention and begin to fail appointments. In doing this, psychologists believe that the boy is overlaying a deeper Freudian fear of bodily mutilation and loss of manhood.

Basic behaviour patterns

It appears that there are three main types of normal children who arrive in the dental surgery.

1. The confident child whose previous experiences in life have left him open to and interested in new experiences.
2. The apprehensive and insecure child whose limited previous experiences in life have been coloured by attitudes learnt from anxious adults but who is capable of being reconditioned with sympathetic management.
3. The emotionally damaged child, fortunately rare, who is suffering from overwhelming fear, perhaps as a result of previously unsympathetic or inadequate treatment, either dental or surgical, or a recent family disaster or other traumatic experience.

The way a child behaves and cooperates in the dental surgery is partly affected by his general lifestyle – family attitudes, friends' experience, general trait towards anxiety and so on – but it is influenced more profoundly and specifically by previous painful experiences during medical or dental treatment, and by prolonged appointments which were beyond the particular child's endurance.

Physically or mentally handicapped children will need special consideration and care based on the advice of the dental surgeon and medical specialist in each individual case.

GENERAL APPROACH

Parents should be encouraged to bring their children to the dental surgery for regular check-ups at 4-monthly intervals from the age of 2 when any possible treatment needs are minimal and simple to carry out while introducing the child to the routines of dentistry.

Reception

The waiting room should have some materials in it that are specially designed for children, which may range from such things as small tables and chairs and large toys such as a rocking horse, to simply an assortment of comic books and papers. These familiar objects will allow a child to identify with his new surroundings more quickly. Whatever is provided should be sturdy, noise-free and inexpensive to replace. Some practices arrange to see all child patients at special sessions and then the waiting room can be specifically arranged for children. Remember that it is often the parent who has to wait there so make sure that there are some grown-up magazines available as well. Early morning appointments are best for young children for they are generally more cooperative when they are not tired or hungry.

The DSA is the first person that the child meets in the dental situation, so make sure that you know his first name readily and that you greet him with a smile, a kind but firm voice and a sympathetic manner. Make sure that his parent gives him the opportunity to visit the toilet before he goes into the surgery. Listen to anything that the parent wants to say about the child's general or dental health and never neglect to tell the dental surgeon about it, particularly any complaint about the teeth that the child has made at home. Try not to discuss possible treatment in front of the child or he may be left with half-understood details for his active imagination to work on. Do not keep children waiting very long, for their ability to cooperate starts to run out from the moment they arrive at the dental surgery whether or not they are receiving treatment. Remember that early treatment sets the pattern of attitude for life and that everyone should strive to make the visits to the dental surgery a routine, almost enjoyable event and not an ordeal to be avoided as long as possible.

Be on the alert for communicable childhood diseases that might possibly be transmitted to other patients. One important example is the simple childhood disease of rubella (German measles) which, if transmitted to a susceptible expectant mother, can severely affect the development of her unborn child.

In the dental surgery
The dental surgeon will decide if a particular parent should accompany the child into the surgery, but usually this is only necessary for very young children, or for a first consultation. The parent should be provided with a seat that does not impede the treatment area of the surgery.

Once the child is in the dental surgery the DSA should continue to maintain a general atmosphere of sympathetic support, but neither she nor the parent must distract the child's attention, either verbally or by their actions, from what the dental surgeon is saying. If all three adults are talking at once, the nervous child will become confused and afraid. The team approach remains important. The chair is adjusted to suit the child and any movement or tilting of the chair announced in advance. Very few child-sized instruments are required for routine dental care and these are generally limited to small handpiece heads and miniature burs, small saliva ejector tips, small diameter cottonwool rolls and small matrix holders.

Treatment should be carried out in an atmosphere of quiet, unhurried and deliberate progress with the minimum of wasted time and effort. Many procedures can be carried out with a minimum of simple instruments to avoid delays. Each new procedure is explained to the child in simple understandable terms and he is warned in advance of noises, tastes and unusual sensations.

Case histories and subsequent treatment planning need the presence of a parent, not only to give a satisfactory account of the child's medical and dental history, but in order that future treatment can be discussed and that parental consent to a course of treatment is obtained. If a general anaesthetic or relative analgesia will be required, the parent or guardian's written consent must be obtained. Consent to local anaesthesia, considered to be a routine treatment procedure, is implied if the parent makes an appointment for their child at the dental surgery, but if possible the parent should be informed that it is to be given. It is always advisable to consult the parent first if any extensive or irreversible treatment such as an extraction or crown preparation is necessary.

Leaving

At the end of the dental visit there is usually a moment or two that can be used to build up a child's confidence for the next appointment. As they leave the surgery the DSA can help by her encouragement, praise and general warm interest. Most children also appreciate a small souvenir: a sticky badge, a painting book, etc. Remember that any child who has had an extraction will want to take home the (well-washed) tooth. Tiny children still believe in the 'tooth fairy' who buys both exfoliated and extracted teeth.

Conservation of the primary teeth

Prevention. It is most important that the parents of young children and older children themselves are taught and motivated to act upon the basic principles of preventive dentistry: diet control, oral hygiene, fluorides, regular dental check-ups.

Early detection of caries. Regular check-ups and, where necessary, radiographic examination (for example, bite-wings) to monitor the teeth.

Treatment of caries

The dental anatomy of the primary teeth has to be taken into account during the treatment of caries and its complications in the primary dentition. The teeth are small and barrel-shaped with thin layers of enamel and dentine overlying a pulp which has long pulp horns extending into the dentine. The root canals of the molars have a complex curved structure and the root apices of all primary teeth lie in close proximity to the forming permanent successors.

Caries in the primary teeth may be treated in three ways:

1. Topical applications of fluorides, in conjunction with renewed efforts at diet control, have been shown to arrest the caries process in early lesions (for example, the use of fluoride varnish (Duraphat).
2. Modification of the shape of the tooth. Overhanging enamel at the margins of cavities may be smoothed away with sandpaper discs and abrasive stones and the cavity 'saucerized' to remove the bulk of caries and to make it self-cleansing in an attempt to stop the carious process.

This means a considerable loss of tooth structure and poor aesthetic appearance. This old method is rarely used nowadays.

3. Restoration of the tooth is the recommended treatment. Using local anaesthesia where necessary all the caries is removed and a cavity is prepared by conventional means so that the tooth may be filled and restored to function and appearance. The cavities are still named using Black's classification, but differ from those prepared in permanent teeth. The preparations have to be shallow to avoid pulpal exposure and are often made wider than in permanent teeth to allow sufficient bulk of material to be inserted to produce a strong restoration. Deep cavities are generally lined with a thin calcium hydroxide cement. In class II restorations a wedged matrix must be used to prevent the production of a cervical overhanging edge. Restoration of the incisor teeth is particularly difficult where the incisal angle has been lost.

Restorative materials for the primary teeth include: silver amalgam; zinc phosphate and carboxylate cements; glass ionomer cements, composite resins and, more rarely, even gold inlays. Very broken-down or weakened teeth can be restored with chrome-steel crowns, either preformed or contoured at the chairside with special pliers. Polycarbonate crowns are available to restore primary incisor teeth in the same way.

Pulp therapy techniques

These can preserve a great many valuable primary teeth that would otherwise have to be extracted long before natural exfoliation should occur, because of pulpal exposure or other pathological condition.

This form of treatment can only be carried out on selected teeth after careful clinical consideration and radiographic examination. The child must be sufficiently cooperative to accept this slightly prolonged type of treatment and should have no general physical or medical contraindication. The numerous techniques vary in detail but fall into the following categories.

Indirect pulp capping. Deep carious lesions approaching pulp exposure can be treated by ensuring that the caries on the floor of the cavity has been reduced to an 'irreducible minimum', and then covering it with a layer of calcium hydroxide cement, before filling the tooth permanently. The result is unpredictable.

Pulp capping. Direct pulp capping of the primary teeth is usually unsuccessful. It can only hope to succeed in the rarely occurring ideal conditions in which the pulp is vital, the exposure small, non-infected and surrounded by non-infected dentine. The exposure is covered with a calcium hydroxide paste, the cavity lined with cement and then filled permanently at the same sitting.

Vital pulpotomy. This is the method of choice with an exposed vital pulp in a primary tooth. Under local anaesthesia and dry, isolated and aseptic conditions the pulp chamber is opened up and its contents removed with a sterile excavator. The amputated ends of the vital pulp tissue remaining in the root canals are then covered with calcium hydroxide paste and the tooth lined and filled permanently.

Devitalizing pulpotomy. If the pulp is vital, but there is evidence of infection in the pulp chamber, the tooth is first prepared as for a vital pulpotomy. Then a pledget of cottonwool moistened with formocresol is placed in the cavity for 2 minutes to sterilize the surface. The pledget is removed and a stiff paste, made up of formocresol, eugenol and zinc oxide powder, is placed in the pulp chamber, and the tooth lined and filled permanently.

Teeth can also be treated in a similar fashion using gluteraldehyde instead of formocresol. Another technique uses paraformaldehyde paste to devitalize the tooth over a period of several days. (Easlick's paste).

Modified pulpectomy and 'root' filling. Where the pulp of a primary tooth is infected and non-vital, extraction of the tooth is usually considered. However, in some cases it is still possible to carry out treatment to prolong its safe retention in the mouth. The disadvantage of this method is that the dental anatomy of the primary molar does not allow thorough mechanical preparation of the root canal in the way that it can be carried out on a permanent tooth. The exposed tooth is opened up widely, the dead pulp tissue is removed to eliminate as much of the infected material as possible and a pledget of cottonwool, soaked in disinfectant such as camphorated monochlorophenol, is firmly sealed into the cavity for 3 or 4 days. If all is well clinically, the tooth is then opened up again, the dressing removed, the pulp chamber filled with a resorbable antiseptic paste and the tooth restored permanently.

In every case of pulp therapy the tooth has to be kept under careful observation both clinically and radiographically and the patient must return immediately should pain, discomfort or swelling occur in the region of the treated tooth.

TRAUMATIC INJURIES TO THE TEETH

Almost 10 per cent of children will damage their teeth in falls, contact sports, street accidents and other mishaps and most of these injuries are to the incisor region of the mouth. Predisposing factors include protruding teeth, slow reaction times to ward off the injury, poor eyesight and a general knockabout, accident-prone disposition. The injury often seems more severe to the parent and the child than it really merits, and prompt and efficient treatment is greatly appreciated by them. Sometimes it is difficult to get the exact story of the accident out of a frightened child, for they tend to minimize a misdemeanour for fear of punishment. It is wise, therefore to look at the whole child first before proceeding to examine the mouth, to make sure that a more severe yet deliberately concealed injury has not taken place that will require urgent medical or hospital attention.

The clinical examination sets out to discover the extent of the injury both to the bones of the skull, face and jaws and to the soft tissues overlying them, particularly the nose and lips. The extent of the loosening or fracture of the teeth is noted and any cuts or tears in the oral mucosa and tongue. Thermal and electrical tests are carried out to determine the extent of the injury to the pulps of the teeth involved. Radiographs are always taken to check for possible injuries to the roots of the teeth and the extent of any displacement from their sockets. Larger films of the skull and jaws may be needed on occasion and sometimes special films of the lip or tongue will reveal that a part of the fractured tooth has been driven into them.

Classification of traumatic injuries to teeth

There are many classifications, some very complex and specialized. The following has been simplified to cover enamel, dentine, pulp, root, and bone and supporting tissues.

1. Fracture of the enamel.
2. Fracture involving the dentine.
3. Fracture exposing the pulp.
4. Fracture of the root.
5. Tooth displaced in the socket.

Treatment

Obviously general care of the injured child, and the arrest of any haemorrhage will take priority. Then the dental treatment may be undertaken; sometimes a tooth is so badly broken that it has to be extracted. Apart from such an emergency, treatment is generally aimed at maintaining the pulp's vitality if possible (or, where this is indicated, taking steps to treat or remove it); at restoring the periodontal attachment as soon as possible after the injury and supporting the tooth until reattachment has taken place; and, finally, restoring the tooth to function and good aesthetic appearance.

Emergency treatment. A tooth that has been completely knocked out must be returned to its socket as quickly as possible if it is to have any chance of recovery. When reimplantation is delayed the avulsed tooth should be placed immediately into the child's moist buccal sulcus or kept submerged in a small quantity of milk. The sharp edges of fractured enamel are smoothed down.

Temporary crown forms filled with sedative cement are put over exposed dentine. Exposed pulps are either treated by capping, vital pulpotomy or pulpectomy. Teeth that have been moved in their sockets are supported using a range of splinting techniques from temporary metal foil cemented over the repositioned tooth to vacuum-formed plastic splints made in the laboratory. They may also be splinted by attaching them to adjacent teeth by an acid-etch technique. Soft tissue wounds are sutured and unsaveable teeth removed. Systemic therapy such as antibiotics or antitetanus treatment is sometimes required for deep, possibly infected wounds.

Semi-permanent treatment. Once the initial healing has taken place, any bruising or swelling has resolved and the final condition of recovery of the pulp and periodontal structure assessed, the semi-permanent treatment can be carried out. This is based on the minimum operative interference with the young growing tissue that will give the maximum function and best aesthetic appearance.

Fractured enamel at the incisal edge can often be ground and contoured at intervals over a period of months until the fractured tooth is an acceptable shape. Loss of more extensive amounts of tooth substance requires restoration, usually with the acid-etch composite technique which has now almost completely superseded the use of faced gold inlays, basket crowns and stainless steel crowns.

Acid-etch technique. The enamel surface of the tooth is etched with acid, and then a composite resin used which polymerizes to mechanically interlock with the roughened surface giving a microstructure bonding and increased retention. This method expands the use of composite materials (for restoring tooth structure so that they may also be used in otherwise non-retentive situations, and for periodontal splinting, temporary retention of orthodontic appliances and covering or veneering malformed teeth.

1. The surface of the tooth is thoroughly cleaned and, where necessary, the fractured enamel margins bevelled with a diamond engine instrument.
2. The tooth is isolated and dried and any exposed dentine protected with a layer of calcium hydroxide cement.
3. The enamel surface is etched where necessary by applying an acid solution for 60 seconds.
4. The tooth is washed thoroughly with water and again dried, when the matt surface of the etched enamel can be seen.
5. Activated enamel bonding resin is applied to the etched surface.
6. The correct shade of composite filling material is mixed and applied over the bonding agent, controlled by a cellulose acetate crown form or matrix.
7. When set, the matrix is removed and the composite restoration finished following the manufacturer's instructions (see p.118).

Splinted teeth. Where a displaced tooth has been splinted it will take a week or two before reattachment will be firm enough to stand occlusal stress; however, the sooner the tooth can be returned to function the better. If the pulp dies during this time the tooth has to be root treated through the surface of the splint.

Where a tooth with a fractured root has been splinted no union between the fragments can occur, and success depends upon the strength of root attachment that can be achieved for the crown-supporting fragment so that the tooth can withstand normal masticatory stresses. In certain cases the root fragments can be splinted permanently by root-filling the tooth with a stainless steel pin.

Extraction. If a traumatized tooth has to be extracted the space may be retained by fitting an immediate denture with the possibility of making a bridge in later years, or the gap may be closed up by orthodontic treatment and the tooth now occupying the space ground or crowned to give a more pleasing appearance.

Permanent treatment. Permanent restoration of these injuries may not be possible until the child has reached its middle teens to allow the teeth and tissues to complete their growth and because some treatment, such as crowns and bridgework, is too time-consuming for a child to tolerate it.

CHAPTER SIXTEEN

Orthodontics

Orthodontics is the branch of dentistry concerned primarily with the prevention or correction of irregularities in position of teeth. It includes the study of the patterns of growth and development of the teeth, jaws and face and also the function of the orofacial soft tissues particularly in swallowing, speech and respiration.

Early diagnosis of irregularities of development of the teeth and jaws is essential if effective treatment is to be carried out in its simplest form. Although some abnormalities will not require or justify treatment, others, if neglected, may upset the quality of the child's life by undermining his future dental health or making him unhappy and self-conscious about his appearance.

Variations in teeth and jaw relationships

The teeth may vary from the normal in *number* (for example, supernumerary or additional teeth, anodontia or the non-development of teeth); in *shape* (for example, gemination or fusion of two teeth, peg-shaped teeth); in *size* or *position* (for example, inclination, rotation, impaction). There may be *crowding* or *spacing* of the teeth. There may be abnormalities of the *arch shape* or the *arch relationship* between the upper and lower jaws.

Definitions

Occlusion means the relationship and contact between the upper and lower teeth upon closure of the jaws.

Normal occlusion occurs when all the teeth are present in the arches and they meet one another in a normal manner.

Malocclusion means abnormal occlusion in which teeth are not in a normal position in relation to adjacent teeth in the same jaw and/or the opposing teeth when the jaws are closed.

Pre-normal occlusion is a malocclusion where the lower teeth meet the upper teeth in front of the normal position.

Post-normal occlusion is where the lower teeth meet the upper teeth behind the normal position.

Overjet is the horizontal overlap of upper over lower incisors.

Overbite is the vertical overlap of upper over lower incisors.

Edge-to-edge bite occurs where there is no overlap and the incisor tips occlude.

Cross-bite occurs when any tooth occludes in the wrong labiolingual position with its opponent, for example, when an upper incisor lies behind a lower incisor, or when the lower arch is wider then the upper.

Open bite is a condition where a space exists between the upper and lower incisor or posterior teeth when the mouth is closed.

Freeway space is the space (approximately 2mm) or clearance between the occlusal surfaces of the teeth when the mandible is in the physiological rest position.

CLASSIFICATIONS OF MALOCCLUSION

There have been many classifications, of which Angle's remains widely accepted.

Angle's classification of malocclusion

Angle (1899) based his classification of dental irregularities on the antero-posterior relationship of the posterior permanent teeth in which the maxillary first permanent molar was regarded as fixed in a constant and normal position, the classification being determined by the relationship of the mandibular molar occluded to it (Fig. 16/1).

Class I. The mandibular arch is in a normal anteroposterior relationship to the maxillary arch. The mesiobuccal cusp of the maxillary first permanent molar occludes with the buccal groove of the mandibular first permanent molar.

Class II. The mandibular arch occludes too far back compared with the maxillary arch.

   Division 1. This occurs when the maxillary incisors are tilted forwards (proclinated).

   Division 2. This occurs when the maxilliary incisors are tilted backwards (retroclinated).

Class III. The mandibular arch occludes too far forward compared with the maxillary arch.

Incisor classification of malocclusion

Some clinicians prefer to describe malocclusion from the incisal relationship when the teeth are in their normal occlusion.

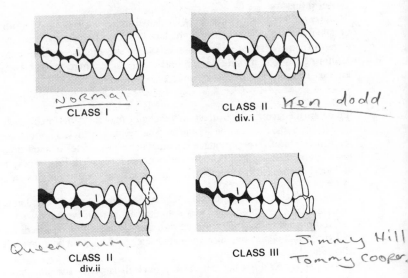

CLASS I ~~NORMAL~~

CLASS II div.i *Ken dodd.*

CLASS II div.ii *Queen mum.*

CLASS III *Jimmy Hill Tommy cooper.*

Fig. 16/1 Angle's classification of malocclusion

Class I. This is when the long axis of the lower incisor crosses the upper through the cingulum of the upper incisor.

Class II. This is when the long axis of the lower incisor crosses the upper behind the cingulum of the upper incisor.

   Division 1. This occurs with the upper incisor overjet increased or proclinated.

   Division 2. This occurs with an increased overbite and reduced overjet or retroclinated.

Class III. This is when the long axis of the lower incisor is anterior to the cingulum of the upper incisor.

CAUSES OF MALOCCLUSION

Positional irregularities of the teeth and the jaw relationship may be caused by general and local factors.

General factors

These can affect the development of the dental arches as a whole and include hereditary factors, the structure of the facial skeleton (skeletal pattern), the form and activity of the facial soft tissues and the size and shape of the teeth. Malformation may include harelip and cleft palate. There may be birth injuries, malnutrition, disease or injury.

Local factors

These are the factors which affect the development of the dental arches only at specific points. For example, bottle feeding, missing teeth, supernumerary teeth, premature loss or prolonged retention of the primary teeth, impaction, loss of permanent teeth, lip and tongue behaviour, thumb or finger sucking and local disease (such as tumours) or injury, may all cause malocclusion.

Diagnosis. Each case requires very full examination because orthodontic problems are often caused by a very complex sequence of events.

A thorough case history is required with special emphasis upon hereditary and congenital factors and also any habits such as thumb-sucking that will affect the shape of the jaws.

The child is examined in the usual way, but with particular attention to the soft tissues of the face and oral cavity (for example, lips and tongue shape and behaviour, swallowing patterns) and the occlusion.

The special examination requires impressions for study models and radiographs. In addition to intraoral films, left and right lateral oblique or orthopantomogram, and occlusal films are generally required to assess the size, root shape and position of unerupted teeth. Specialist orthodontists may also require a standard position lateral skull radiograph for *cephalometric analysis* of the skeletal pattern to be made by measuring certain planes, lines and angles between standard reference points on the skull.

When all this information is available, the orthodontist can complete his diagnosis and make a treatment plan. This must be discussed in detail with the child and his parents so that their full cooperation and consent is assured before long-term treatment is started.

Indications for treatment

Orthodontic treatment is indicated in cases where the present and future function, appearance and health of the orofacial structure is affected:

1. When the abnormality interferes with masticatory function or speech.
2. Where the aesthetic appearance is poor.
3. Where the malposition or malocclusion predisposes towards caries, periodontal disease or temporomandibular joint disorders.
4. Where the abnormality may increase the risk of root resorption, tooth impaction or accidental trauma to the teeth.

5. Where good cooperation and interest from the patient and his parents are to be expected.

METHODS OF TREATMENT

Basically, orthodontic treatment falls into the following four categories.

Elimination of causative habits

This can be done by reasoning with the older child and perhaps constructing a simple appliance to help him to break the habit. Habits such as thumb-sucking in the mixed dentition period have a deep psychological basis and treatment should be aimed at the cause rather than the outward habit itself.

Operative treatment

1. By extracting teeth to relieve crowding or by the extraction of retained deciduous teeth where they impede normal eruption.
2. By selective grinding, which can sometimes allow a tooth to move into the correct place.
3. By surgically exposing or repositioning unerupted teeth, for example, canines.
4. By operating on the soft tissues, for example, fraenectomy (where the fraenum is the cause of a space between teeth) or bone, for example, altering the position of sectors of teeth and alveolus, or altering the contour of the mandible.

Appliances

The bone supporting the teeth is a living substance that reacts to the forces placed upon it by muscular and other stresses. Teeth and groups of teeth can be moved into new positions by the use of continual pressure sufficient to cause the bone to be remodelled. These changes can be achieved more rapidly in growing children and young people. The pressure upon the teeth must not exceed certain limits or the vitality of the tooth and the adjacent periodontal membrane may be affected. In appliance therapy the pressure must be applied accurately and be under complete control while based on a firm anchorage. This *anchorage* may be gained by the use of a removable plate or a fixed metal appliance attached to groups of teeth, or from an extraoral anchorage such as a webbing cap to which wires from the mouth can be attached.

Active appliances. These exert pressure on the teeth to be moved and must be kept under frequent revision by the dental surgeon. The pressure may be continuous, as with metal springs or elastic bands, or it may be intermittent, as when small screw systems are incorporated into the appliance and turned at intervals to 'wedge' the tooth or group of teeth into position.

Passive appliances. These do not exert a pressure and are used to retain teeth in a desired position at certain stages of treatment.

Functional appliances. These alter the environment of the teeth and employ orofacial muscle forces to induce tooth movement.

Fixed appliances. Stainless steel bands are cemented onto posterior teeth and steel brackets are bonded to anterior teeth in order that arch wires, springs, etc. can be attached to them. These appliances can exert a continuous effect upon the teeth and thus, although they have a poor appearance and are hard to keep clean, the desired effect is obtained quickly. Fixed appliances are able to move teeth in all three planes and can therefore carry out the full range of orthodontic tooth movements.

Removable appliances. These are usually constructed of acrylic with stainless steel arch wires, clasps and springs. Being removable they allow normal oral hygiene procedures and can be taken out for adjustment at intervals. In certain cases they need to be worn only at night. A removable appliance can easily be lost, damaged or forgotten by the patient.

  Norwegian plate. Also called the Andresen appliance or Monobloc, this is constructed to act as a functional appliance. It uses muscular power to reposition teeth as it directs their movement and eruption. The single acrylic plate is fitted to both arches and draws the mandible into the desired position as well as producing and directing forces upon individual and groups of teeth.
  Frankel appliance. This consists of a series of acrylic flanges joined by a stainless steel wire framework. Like the Andresen, this appliance contacts both upper and lower teeth at the same time and is generally worn only at night.
  (A wide range of orthodontic pliers is available for use in the construction, contouring and adjustment of the metal wires and tapes of various dimensions that are used in most appliances).

In all cases the patient and the parent should be carefully instructed about the use and care of the orthodontic appliance. For example, some appliances need daily home adjustment of screws while others require the attachment of elastic bands, head gear, etc.
  The patient is seen at regular intervals during treatment:

1. To observe the progress of the treatment.
2. To ensure and reinforce the patient's continuing cooperation and motivation.
3. To monitor the appliance and make adjustments and repairs.
4. To ensure the maintenance of a high standard of oral hygiene.
5. To ensure that the teeth are caries-free and the periodontal condition is healthy.

CHAPTER SEVENTEEN

Preventive Dentistry

Preventive dentistry is the science and practice of measures to prevent the onset of diseases of the teeth and neighbouring soft tissues.

The commonest dental diseases are dental caries and the periodontal diseases and, to a very great extent, they can be prevented, halted or their effects minimized if appropriate action is taken early enough.

By tradition the dental surgeon and his patient have been almost completely preoccupied by the practical problems of treating the effects of already established dental disease. One course of treatment inevitably followed the next. It is only in recent years that real progress has been made in changing their attitudes so that an effort is also made to preserve an existing healthy state by taking definite action.

DENTAL EPIDEMIOLOGY

The science of *dental epidemiology* is concerned with investigating the distribution of dental disease within a population to allow analysis of the cause and of the best methods of its treatment and prevention. It requires great precision and skill and uses many standard indices of assessment, such as the DMF count (decayed, missing, filled teeth).

The *incidence* of a disease indicates the number of occurrences of a disease over a given period of time, while the *prevalence* shows the number of cases in a population on that day.

Recent surveys have shown a decline in the prevalence of dental caries of 30–50 per cent in 20 years in developed countries while the percentage in developing countries is rising (perhaps due to increased access to sugar, etc.).

THE CAUSES OF PERIODONTAL DISEASE AND DENTAL CARIES

Both these diseases are caused initially when dental plaque is allowed to form on the surfaces of erupted teeth. Its extensive presence indicates a poor standard of oral hygiene.

Dental plaque
Dental plaque forms initially as a cell-free pellicle or film which soon matures to become an adherent layer, containing organic material, mucin from saliva, desquamated (loosened) epithelial cells and food debris, colonized by various bacteria and micro-organisms (*Streptoccocus mutans*, lactobacilli, spirochaetes, actinomyces and others). It forms initially in pits and fissures, between the teeth and at the gingival margins.

Gingivitis and periodontal disease
Gingivitis and periodontal disease begin because the gingival plaque bacteria produce substances which cause gum inflammation. Later the gingival and subgingival plaque can mineralize to form calculus.

Dental caries
Dental caries is a multifactorial disease. In simple terms certain bacteria found in dental plaque can ferment carbohydrates (such as sugars) to produce an acid strong enough to demineralize susceptible tooth substance within a few minutes.
   Thus four factors are involved:

1. The presence of dental plaque because of the acid-producing bacteria.
2. The presence of fermentable carbohydrates in the diet.
3. A susceptible tooth.
4. Sufficient time for the carious demineralization to occur.

PREVENTION OF PERIODONTAL DISEASE AND DENTAL CARIES

It is convenient to list the methods of preventing both periodontal disease and dental caries together because general oral hygiene techniques can tackle both problems at the same time.

Dental plaque
Although it is impossible to remove dental plaque totally from the teeth and gum margins, much can be done to reduce its presence and to counteract its effects.

By improving oral hygiene. This is particularly important in the prevention of periodontal disease.

   Tooth brushing. This should be carried out regularly at least after breakfast and last thing at night. Generally, the toothbrush should have a short head, a flat bristle surface and a firm non-bending handle. The bristles should be of medium hard nylon (unless another hardness is recommended by the dental surgeon) and must be allowed to dry out completely after each period of use or they will become softened and unsuitable for the task.

Toothbrushing techniques have to be adapted to suit each individual's mouth. The methods of brushing an intact arch will differ from those where several teeth have been lost or for a child in the mixed dentition stage. Parents must brush their children's teeth themselves, or finish it off, or supervise the procedure depending on the child's age, at least once a day.

Brushing back and forth in a mesiodistal direction is bad both for the gingivae and the damaging effect it will have on the thin enamel that covers the necks of the teeth. Many different techniques for brushing the teeth have been recommended. One method recommended for general use is the circular scrub where the bristles are placed against a segment of teeth with the bristles at an angle of 45° to the tooth surface and the tips of the bristles carried into the spaces between the teeth and the gums; the brush head is then moved in a circular path to clean that segment before moving to the next. Another method is to brush the teeth the way they grow, from the gingival margin to the tip of the tooth, using sweeping strokes. This action must be repeated both on the buccal and labial surfaces and on the lingual and palatal surfaces taking great care not to miss an area. After this the biting surfaces should be brushed thoroughly, and finally the loosened particles of food debris should be rinsed out of the mouth with plenty of water. Thorough toothbrushing will be easier if it is carried out while looking in a mirror to check the results visually. A most effective aid to ensure good oral hygiene is the *disclosing solution* or tablet which is introduced into the mouth before brushing commences and colours all food debris and plaque bright red. The teeth are then to be brushed by an approved method until all the stained material has been removed.

Single-tufted, or interspace toothbrushes can be used for stimulating small areas of gingivae between particular teeth or for cleaning otherwise inaccessible areas of the mouth, such as around fixed bridgework.

Mains and battery-powered electric toothbrushes can be used to clean the teeth very thoroughly and quickly with the minimum of effort and require little manual dexterity to manipulate them into various places in the mouth.

Interdental cleaning. The spaces between the teeth usually cannot be reached by the bristles of a conventional toothbrush. Trapped food particles and plaque may be cleaned from the interdental space by sliding a length of *dental floss* carefully between the teeth and then moving it gently up and down, pressing it first against one tooth and then the other. This method is particularly useful for dislodging fragments of fibrous food such as meat or apple skin that have become wedged between the teeth.

Another method involves the use of specially shaped *wood points*. These are made of firm or soft wood and the patient must be advised which is suitable for his personal use. They are only to be used where the interdental papillae do not fill the interdental space in a healthy mouth. The wood point is passed gently between the teeth, low down at gingival level and moved back and forth to dislodge food debris and at the same time massage the interdental papilla to stimulate and harden the otherwise inaccessible epithelial surface.

Water can be used in an attempt to wash bulky food debris from between the teeth but cannot, of course, remove dental plaque. A small quantity is taken into the mouth, forced repeatedly between the tongue and the cheek via the interdental spaces and then swallowed or spat out. *Oral irrigation* machines are available that produce a strong, pulsating jet of water or mouthwash through a fine nozzle that can be directed against the surface of the teeth and through the interdental space with considerable cleansing effect.

Dentrifrices (aids to cleaning teeth with a brush). Toothpastes help to remove plaque by their mild abrasive and detergent action. Their pleasant taste encourages good oral hygiene habits. In addition they usually contain fluoride which becomes concentrated in plaque and seems to affect its bacterial activity. The fluoride may also be absorbed onto the surface of the tooth enamel and make it more resistant to acid and to new plaque formation. The increased use of fluoride toothpastes has been linked with the recently reported decline in caries prevalence in developed countries.

Chemical and antibacterial agents. Surface active agents are being sought to repel the attachment of plaque to the teeth. Antibacterial agents such as 0.2 per cent chlorhexidine solution mouthwashes or gel application twice a day have been shown to reduce plaque formation.

Immunization. Research into possible immunization methods against the organisms that cause dental caries continues to attract interest but as yet is confined to experimental animals.

Diet control

This may be used to reduce the acid-producing effects of bacterial activity within the plaque when sugars are present in the mouth.

The acid is produced within a few minutes and it takes about 15 to 20 minutes for the diluting and neutralizing effects of saliva to take effect and start to counteract it.

All sugary food and drink containing fermentable carbohydrates represent a danger to the teeth, not related to the quantity of sugary material consumed as much as the frequency and duration of time that the teeth are exposed to it.

Bottle-fed babies should be weaned gradually to drinking from a cup by the time they are 1 year old, otherwise the sweetened milk, vitamin syrups and fruit juices that trickle slowly over the newly erupted primary teeth will result in rampant caries within a few months. This will particularly affect the teeth of the older child who is 'got off to sleep' with a 'propped' bottle in the pram or cot, or who is comforted and quietened during the day with a dummy or pacifier dipped in jam or syrup, or has a longer-acting reservoir pacifier containing sugary solutions. The same danger arises with sugary medicines, especially when they are given at night. Parents should be made aware of these dangers to an infant's teeth.

Ideally, everyone should eat ample well-balanced meals at regular intervals and thus not require the between-meals snacks that can be so damaging to the teeth. If possible a meal should be finished off with a savoury food to counteract the sugar's acid-forming effects in the plaque. The child who has an unlimited quantity of sweets and spends much of his waking day with one slowly dissolving in his mouth, or the man who is trying to give up smoking and seeks an alternative oral pacification of his psychological stresses by an endless series of peppermints are both running a high risk of rampant caries.

It is hard to deprive children of sweets altogether, particularly in the face of constant persuasive advertising techniques to sell them. An alternative to prohibition has been suggested; the child may have one sweet-eating orgy a week, say Saturday afternoon, when he may eat as many sweets as he wishes for the limited period.

However, he should first clean his teeth to remove the waiting plaque and afterwards follow this dentally hazardous escapade by very thorough and vigorous oral hygiene. At all other times, any craving between meals should be satisfied with cheese, fruit, nuts (*not advisable for children who have a small windpipe and can easily choke on one*), potato crisps and other attractive food products that are not caries-promoting.

The importance of diet control can be emphasized by arranging for the patient or the child's parent to keep a 3-day record of all food and drink consumed plus times and amounts, preferably including one weekend day. Subsequent discussion about this record with the dental surgeon, as he/she checks to identify sugary foods and recommend acceptable non-sugary alternatives, will do much to bring the whole matter to the level of conscious thought and choice in future.

Watch out for confectionery, acid or sweet fruit juices. Cut out sugar in tea, coffee, cocoa, etc. Check the sugar content of prepared foods, for example, baked beans (4 per cent sugar), tomato ketchup (22 per cent), boiled sweets (98 per cent), etc.

The tooth

Development. A great deal has been written about the importance of vitamins, balanced diets, etc., but little evidence has been found to relate nutrition during tooth development to final tooth structure apart from the benefits of fluoride. However, hereditary disorders of formation or disturbances of the tooth environment, for example, in fevers and local inflammation, can upset the processes of tooth development and mineralization so that teeth erupt with vulnerable and ill-formed (hypoplastic) enamel.

Fluorides. It has been discovered that if a minute trace of the element fluorine is available to the child's body during the period that the teeth are formed and mineralized, then the enamel formed is stronger and more resistant to dental caries. In some parts of the world fluorides are present naturally in the drinking water and it has been shown that people born and bred there have a much lower caries rate than average. Excessive amounts of fluoride, on the other hand, can upset the normal formation of the enamel with resultant mottling of the teeth. It is known that one part per million of fluoride in the drinking water is the best for partial control of dental caries. It is suggested that some 55 to 60 per cent reduction is achieved in this way. Where water supplies have not been fluoridated, tablets containing fluoride can be taken every day during the period of tooth formation with possibly a 50 per cent reduction of caries. Topical application of fluoride to erupted teeth in the form of freshly made up solutions or in a gel or lacquer can give a 20 to 30 per cent reduction, while the daily use of a toothpaste containing fluorides or rinsing the mouth with a very dilute solution can give a caries reduction of 20 to 30 per cent. Sometimes a combination of internal and topical use of fluoride can be suggested as a doubly effective method of gaining this benefit.

Fissure sealants. Plastic materials have been developed which may be used to seal pits and fissures of non-carious teeth for long periods and thus eliminate potential danger spots where plaque can collect undisturbed.

Sealants may be of filled or unfilled resins, come in different colours and may either be chemically cured or light-cured.

1. The teeth to be treated are cleaned with an oil-free, non-fluoride polishing paste and washed thoroughly.
2. A quadrant of teeth is isolated with cottonwool rolls (or rubber dam) and the teeth thoroughly dried with the air syringe.
3. The etching solution is applied to the surfaces with a cottonwool pledget for 60 seconds.
4. The teeth are washed thoroughly (carefully avoiding saliva contamination), the tooth dried with air, and new cottonwool rolls placed in position. The etched surfaces will appear to be whitened and frosty.

5. The selected resin is prepared according to the manufacturer's instructions and applied to the tooth fissures.
6. After about 2 minutes the resin has set, and is checked for coverage, retention and occlusion with the opposing teeth before the patient is dismissed.

Every sealed surface should be re-examined at 6-monthly intervals and resealed if necessary.

Time factors

Dental caries in its earliest stages can be reversible. If the acid-producing process is stopped, its effect on decalcification of the enamel surface will be reversed by the buffering effect (change resistant) of the saliva and remineralization can take place from salts in the saliva. This underlines the importance of reducing the time that sugars are present in the mouth. Thus the ebb and flow effect of dissolution and repair of the enamel will be overbalanced over a period of weeks or months to proceed to cavity formation if the acid periods are longer than the recovery periods.

Periodontal disease is also affected by the time that gingival plaque is allowed to remain undisturbed. If it is left for a few days it will become calcified into calculus. Daily removal of the plaque by careful toothbrushing and interdental cleaning is essential.

MONITORING

In order that oral health be maintained the patient's mouth must be examined at regular intervals. From past experience this has always been done at 6-monthly intervals – but of course this period must be shorter for dental disease-prone people and perhaps lengthier for individuals who have been proved to have good oral hygiene and to have sound motivation to take care of themselves. Nevertheless, once a patient has been brought to a state of dental health, his name should be placed on a recall list or at least he should be advised to seek a further inspection after the recommended interval. These regular dental check-ups are a sound principle of preventive dentistry for they mean that any carious lesions, periodontal disorders, etc., are discovered early before they can deteriorate. This will ensure that any treatment needed is minimal and simple to carry out and thus visits to the dental surgery remain pleasant, acceptable and unlikely to cause fear and apprehension.

Monitoring for caries includes careful examination of all the surfaces of the teeth in a good light, with the teeth dried.

Probing the teeth has to be done with care in case the chalky demineralized surface, the first stage of caries, is damaged and broken by the probe itself before it has had a chance to remineralize (perhaps assisted by diet control and topical fluoride.) The teeth can also be examined both radiographically and with a fibreoptic light. New diagnostic methods are constantly being sought and there have recently been experiments to detect caries by changes of electrical conductivity, as yet with varying success.

The gingival and periodontal condition is also monitored using indices of inflammation, plaque scores and graduated periodontal pocket depth probes.

PREVENTIVE RESTORATIONS

Where a molar tooth has a stained or compromised fissure then there is a danger of 'occult' caries occurring. Even with adequate radiographs this is sometimes difficult to diagnose decisively. Then, instead of the 'give prevention time to work' policy, many operators suggest 'if in doubt investigate'. The tiny stained fissure is explored with a minimal-sized bur. If the pit or fissure does not penetrate the enamel, the fissure is then filled with composite and the tooth fissure sealed over the top of it. If the cavity is found to have penetrated as far as the dentine, then the carious dentine is removed, the cavity lined, filled with composite and, if appropriate, the tooth fissure sealed as before.

DENTAL HEALTH EDUCATION

The Health Education Authority says that dental health educators can confidently restrict their advice to four simple messages:

1. Insist on water fluoridation.
2. Restrict food and drink containing sugar to mealtimes.
3. Clean the teeth and gums thoroughly every day.
4. Use a fluoride toothpaste.

The simple basic facts about methods of preventing dental disease must continually be made available to all levels of the public. Adults have to be made aware of them both for themselves and in their capacity as parents and examples to young people. Mothers and expectant mothers have a particularly important role in this respect.

All people working in health and education services, for example, medical practitioners, welfare workers, nurses and schoolteachers, should be kept up to date with the latest facts about dental health matters so that they can pass on the information, at appropriate times, during their contact with the public.

Every member of the dental team has an individual duty to communicate this information, with *the direct supervision and permission of the dental surgeon*, with almost missionary zeal. The basic facts are very simple. The real problem is how to motivate people to take notice and act upon the knowledge. No-one in the dental team must neglect an opportunity to teach people, either as individuals or in groups of children or adults, about the importance of having a healthy mouth and the methods of gaining and maintaining it. A great deal of attractive teaching aids and materials in the form of pamphlets and books, posters, film strips, tape-slides and lecture notes, teaching models, sound movie films and so on, are readily available from the professional organizations (e.g. the General Dental Council, Health Education Authority, and so on). With such inspiring and motivating material to hand, no one need hesitate about their ability to pass on the message of dental health.

OTHER ASPECTS OF PREVENTIVE DENTISTRY

Preventive dentistry is not solely concerned with the problems of dental caries and the periodontal diseases. This attitude of prediction of events and the institution of corrective measures to achieve and maintain a healthy situation must also be brought to all other aspects of dentistry. For example, in children's dentistry irregularities of growth must be detected and forecast early so that simple corrective measures can be started and thus prevent more serious problems later on. The increasing use of mouthguards in contact sports has emphasized the value of these plastic devices in the avoidance of fractured or dislocated teeth. In prosthetics, the patient fitted with satisfactory full dentures is encouraged to return to have them checked at least every 2 years so that changes in the bite or damage to the oral mucosa due to loss of fit can be prevented. In the surgery, care with x-ray radiation, the reduction of possible mercury fumes, the precautions to avoid transference of infection, and so on, are all preventive measures in themselves.

CHAPTER EIGHTEEN

Hazards and Emergencies in the Dental Surgery

When a patient comes into the dental surgery the full responsibility for his safety and well-being is in the hands of the dental surgeon and his staff. Potential hazards, both in the environment and in treatment, must be anticipated and where possible eliminated. It is better to foresee and avoid emergencies than to have to deal with them.

THE HEALTH AND SAFETY AT WORK etc ACT 1974

This act emphasizes the legal responsibility borne by employers and staff to reduce the likelihood of accidental injury or health risks at their place of work to themselves, or members of the general public (patients, for example), in relation to work activities. This legislation introduces penalties for failing to maintain safe standards; although Codes of Practice are being drawn up by the Health and Safety Commission, everyone should be aware of the need to review current practices in the light of these legal requirements. It is quite impossible to list every potential hazard, but it is stressed that it is the personal responsibility of every member of the dental team to protect himself and others.

For example, fire precautions on the premises must be checked regularly and members of the staff made fully aware of the exits in case of fire, and the positioning of fire extinguishers, etc. Exits must be kept clear at all times, extinguishers must be regularly maintained and all staff trained how to use them.

Any accident or defect in equipment, supplies, fixture and fittings must be reported immediately to the head of the team, and steps take at once to prevent a recurrence of the incident. All accidents to patients or staff must be recorded in the accident book, and should include date, time and names of staff present, to whom reported and action taken. Such records have to be kept for a minimum period of 7 years.

For specific risks see Chapter 7 (radiological hazards); Chapter 8 (mercury contamination); and Chapter 12 (anaesthetic hazards).

GENERAL HAZARDS

The following cannot be comprehensive, but the examples given will show the basic preventive attitude that must be adopted by the dental team.

Furniture and fittings

Are there any unfastened linoleum or carpet edges, polished or uneven floor surfaces, loose mats or electrical cables which may cause the patient to trip, slip and fall? Are the stairs adequately lit? Are there any projecting corners of desks, shelves or cabinets that the unwary patient might knock himself against?

In all respects every member of the dental team has a responsibility and obligation to be alert to discover and take adequate steps to deal with any hazards that may put their own or other people's health and safety at risk.

Patient

Is there anything about him/her that will require special care and consideration? This may perhaps be a physical limitation: blindness, poor eyesight, deafness, unsteadiness on the feet or a medical condition. It may be emotional or mental instability leading to poor cooperation during treatment or a tendency to make sudden, uncontrolled movements. All visitors to the surgery must be protected as well as the patient; for example, a child should not be left unattended or allowed to run about the surgery while another member of the family is being treated.

Dental equipment

This must be maintained in reliable working order so that there is no likelihood of it breaking down during treatment with resultant danger to the patient.

Electricity must be treated with respect and a constant watch kept on electric cables, wiring and plugs to avoid the possibility of electric shocks due to worn wiring or inadequately earthed equipment.

Heat is a constant hazard in the surgery. The patient must sometimes be warned about, and always protected from, gas flames, sterilizers and autoclaves. Instruments should never be 'flamed' with burning alcohol. If alcohol or other inflammable liquids are used at the chairside they should be dispensed in small quantities in a container that is kept well away from any naked flame. *Never* put stock bottles of these liquids on the bracket table.

X-ray apparatus must be used and maintained with adequate precautions (see Chapter 7).

Instruments and materials. Very rarely an instrument such as a bur or a reamer may break while being used in the patient's mouth. This danger can be minimized if care is taken to avoid weakening such instruments during sterilization and general handling and to replace them frequently with new ones. When a breakage occurs, all the fragments must be traced and recovered, sometimes a time-consuming and worrying matter.

The patient must be protected against the common accident of dropping instruments or materials on to him. His clothes must be covered with adequate bibs and towels for the particular operation undertaken and instruments, drugs and materials should not be passed to the dental surgeon over the patient's face. Where the patient is lying flat his eyes should be protected with goggles.

All instruments must be properly sterilized to avoid the hazard of cross-infection. All drugs must be properly and clearly labelled to prevent mistakes in their use.

Consent to treatment

This must be obtained from the patient or, in the case of a minor under the age of 16, from his parent or responsible guardian. This consent must be in writing when a general anaesthetic is to be used. The DSA should be present in the surgery at all times during dental treatment as both witness and chaperone.

TREATMENT HAZARDS

Most hazards will be avoided when an adequate and thorough case history has been taken at the start of a course of treatment so that the patient's general health and medical condition are known. It is particularly important to know if the patient is receiving medical treatment and drugs for any reason, and further up-to-date information must be sought from the patient each time an anaesthetic or other drug is given. Before a general anaesthetic is given always check that the patient has followed the instruction about not eating or drinking for the previous 4 hours.

The prevention of local complications during treatment is entirely the dental surgeon's responsibility, but the DSA must be aware of the potential hazards such as slips and cuts with sharp instruments and damage to anaesthetized parts. The patient must always be protected from the danger of swallowing or inhaling small instruments, by using, for example, a rubber dam or by anchoring the instrument with a length of dental floss.

During treatment or in the immediate postoperative period the patient may suffer haemorrhage, collapse or loss of consciousness and the treatment of these emergencies is described on pages 216–21.

Postoperative care

As soon as treatment is completed everything must be done to ensure that nothing untoward occurs during the postoperative recovery period. Patients will need time to recover themselves before being allowed to leave. Those who have had a sedative drug, an anaesthetic or prolonged treatment, may have to spend time in the recovery room and may not be fit to go home unless accompanied by a responsible adult. Patients under the influence of drugs must not be allowed to take part in any potentially hazardous activity such as driving themselves home by car or finding their own way home by public transport.

Any postoperative instructions about what to do in the event of pain, haemorrhage or infection together with the follow-up appointment should be given to the patient in writing so that he may study them later.

The DSA must confirm that all bleeding has ceased before allowing the patient to leave after an extraction.

CONDITIONS REQUIRING SPECIAL PRECAUTIONS

AIDS (acquired immune deficiency syndrome)

This disease is the consequence of infection by the blood-borne virus HIV (human immunodeficiency virus). Infection with HIV does *not* mean that AIDS will develop. The virus itself is delicate and has a low infectivity and is not resistant to heat or chemical disinfectants. It appears that the disease is transmitted via the body fluids, particularly semen and blood, and plasma products. At present the majority of cases are found in homosexual/bisexual men, intravenous drug abusers, patients treated with unscreened blood products and infants born to infected mothers. AIDS leaves the patient vulnerable to opportunistic diseases which in turn may result in specific lung infections, fungal, bacterial and virus infections and certain cancers, such as Kaposi's sarcoma. The infection can be detected by a specific HIV antibody test.

Information that a patient suffers from AIDS or is an HIV carrier must be regarded as strictly confidential. Identified AIDS patients requiring dental treatment need to be cared for from a basis of sympathetic understanding; although it appears to be unlikely that alerted health care workers will contract the disease from these patients, *every precaution to protect the members of the team and other patients must be observed.*

Anaphylactic shock

Drug sensitivity reactions can vary from mild skin rashes to severe anaphylactic shock where the patient who has been sensitized by a previous dose of a drug suffers a serious reaction to a second dose of the same drug. He feels weak and nauseated, rapidly becomes pale and loses consciousness; the sudden fall in blood pressure causes a weak pulse. He may also suffer convulsions, total collapse and even death unless immediate treatment is given.

The patient must be laid flat and the legs elevated to restore the blood pressure. Adrenaline (1:1000) 0.5ml is injected intramuscularly and oxygen given. An injection containing 100mg of hydrocortisone sodium succinate should be given intramuscularly. (*Note*: The DSA is *not* qualified to give an injection to a patient.)

Penicillin sensitivity is one potential cause of this wide range of reactions.

Bleeding tendency

This may be *hereditary*, for example, haemophilia, or *acquired*, for example, through anticoagulants, or in leukaemia or thrombocytopenia (white cell or platelet disorders). Patients with a history of prolonged bleeding, for more than 36 hours, need to have their blood investigated and screened before any surgery or deep injections are carried out.

Anticoagulants. Patients who have suffered disorders causing thrombosis (blood clots in the blood vessels) are given anticoagulant drugs to prevent further clot formation or embolus (clot fragments escaping into the general circulation). For example, a patient who has had a coronary thrombosis (heart attack) will be treated in this way. Any dental treatment, such as extractions, for such a patient will probably result in prolonged and dangerous bleeding that will require admission to hospital. This can be avoided by obtaining an adequate drug history *before* commencing treatment, and these patients usually carry a card explaining their drug regimen. Extractions can only be carried out safely after a period in which the anticoagulant drug dose is adjusted under a doctor's supervision, and the clotting time has returned to acceptable limits.

Corticosteroid treatment

A number of medical conditions such as rheumatoid arthritis, skin and eye diseases are treated with steroid hormones. These drugs, taken over long periods, can leave the patient liable to collapse as a result of stress unless the steroid hormone dosage has been specially adjusted before a dental operation. Such patients usually carry a special medical card which should be shown to the dental surgeon. If a patient collapses in the dental surgery due to this problem he should be admitted to hospital. Emergency treatment, after consultation with a doctor, involves the administration of hydrocortisone sodium succinate. Steroid hormones lead to delay in wound healing.

Diabetes

Diabetic patients have difficulty in controlling their blood sugar levels due to a hormone (insulin) deficiency. If these levels are not adequately balanced by special diet precautions and/or the use of insulin, problems of *ketosis* (upset carbohydrate metabolism, detected by breath smelling of alcohol, gradually leading to a coma), or *hypoglycaemia* can arise. Patients suffering hypoglycae-mia (a lack of blood sugar), feel weak and hungry, become anxious, sweat, and may lose consciousness. Special precautions must be taken to maintain blood sugar levels during certain dental treatments, such as general anaes-thesia and multiple extractions, and also in the presence of dental infections. These patients are usually treated only after consultation with their doctor.

Drugs
Always remember that a high proportion of patients are taking tablets and medicines, both of the prescribed and 'over-the-counter' kind. Many of these drugs will have important implications in the dental surgery because of possible side-effects and because their use is an indicator of illness. The patient's records must be constantly updated in this respect.

Epilepsy
There is usually a history of previous epileptic attacks. The patient may experience an aura that warns him of an impending attack and then fall unconscious usually with convulsions. Treatment is directed towards pro-tecting the patient from injuring himself in falling and also protecting the tongue from being bitten, until he recovers consciousness. Epilepsy may be controlled by the patient taking antiepileptic drugs over long periods: gingival hypoplasia is a side-effect of *phenytoin*.

Heart disease
Cardiac disease is common and these patients require special attention. They can be affected adversely by pain and anxiety, and should avoid general anaesthesia. They may be taking anticoagulants.

Angina. This severe pain behind the sternum is caused by a spasm of the arteries serving the heart muscle, and may be brought on by overactivity or stress. It usually lasts only a few minutes and can be relieved by the patient placing a glyceryl trinitrate tablet under the tongue. Patients suffering from angina should only be treated after consultation with their doctor.

Cardiac infarction (coronary thrombosis). This occurs when a blood clot or thrombus blocks one of the main end-arteries serving the muscle of the heart. There is a sudden onset of prolonged severe pain behind the sternum, perhaps radiating to the left arm and neck. The patient looks grey-faced and shocked. An ambulance should be called for immediately. The patient should remain undisturbed, lying down where possible and kept warm. Oxygen may be given. Morphine for the pain and intensive care in hospital are urgently required.

Heart lesions. Patients with heart lesions (for example, heart murmurs, damaged heart valves or a history of rheumatic fever) require antibiotic cover during dental surgical treatment to prevent possible complications due to stray organisms released into the bloodstream. The precise regimen is usually advised by the patient's doctor, but penicillin or one of its derivatives (in penicillin-sensitive patients, erythromycin) is given orally to the patient about an hour before the operation, and may need to be continued over the next 24 hours. Patients who have prosthetic heart valves also require this kind of prophylaxis.

Patients who have had cardiac pacemakers fitted require special care because, very rarely, the pacemaker's action may be affected by certain electrical or ultrasonic instruments in the dental surgery.

Hepatitis B

This is an inflammatory disease of the liver. It is caused by the hepatitis B virus (HBV), a sturdy and highly infectious virus which is very resistant to boiling water and antiseptics and is only killed by hypochlorite solutions or autoclaving. HBV can live outside the body for several weeks. Hepatitis B has a 1 per cent mortality rate in hospitalized cases and is a major cause of liver cancer and chronic liver disease. About 50 per cent of cases are subclinical (not noticed or diagnosed), and some 10 per cent of cases retain the virus after recovery and become carriers. Diagnosis is made by a blood test. Transmission is by blood and body fluids and by needlestick injuries; thus dental treatment is a *potential source of infection.* Health care workers are at risk. All dental clinical staff should be vaccinated against the disease (three injections at 0, 1 and 6 month intervals and with a booster after a further 5 years).

Pregnancy

The normal expectant mother requires special consideration. Her treatment is best undertaken during the middle 3 months of her pregnancy and she must not be kept in the dental chair for long periods. Her comfortable positioning is important and oxygen should be available in the surgery should she faint, to prevent danger to the baby. The taking of radiographs must be kept to a minimum because x-rays can affect the fetus adversely. The expectant mother should only be given drugs for good reasons, because they can pass through the placenta and affect the fetus or later pass into the mother's milk and affect the infant.

Respiratory disease

Even simple respiratory diseases such as the common cold are contraindications to general anaesthesia because of the likelihood of postoperative pulmonary (lung) complications. Patients with more severe lung diseases must not be given drugs such as sedatives which will depress respiration.

Sickle-cell anaemia and sickle-cell trait

This is an inherited disease which is confined almost entirely to the negro races, although cases are found occasionally in people from Mediterranean countries and Asia.

Abnormal haemoglobin in the red cells causes them to assume a sickle shape at low oxygen tensions with increased blood viscosity and possible capillary thrombosis; such changes may cause risk to life. Any patients who may be thought to fall into this group should have had a blood test to ascertain whether they have the condition before they are given a general anaesthetic (Sickledex test).

EMERGENCIES

HAEMORRHAGE

This is the escape of blood from the blood vessels, and may be *primary* when it occurs at the time of the injury, or during surgery, due to the cutting of blood vessels; *reactionary* when it occurs after the blood pressure is reduced during a period of shock after an injury, and rises again; or *secondary* when it occurs as a result of infection of the wound and break down of the vessels before permanent repair has taken place, usually 7 to 10 days later. The bleeding may be *arterial*, from a severed artery, when the blood is bright red and spurts in pulsating jets; *venous*, from a cut vein, when the blood is dark red or purple and flows continuously; or *capillary*, from the minute peripheral vessels, when the blood is red and oozes steadily but is not copious. The average healthy male can lose 570–850ml ($1-1\frac{1}{2}$ pints) and only feel weak, whereas a sick or elderly person or a child may suffer considerably from the loss of a much smaller amount.

Temporary arrest of haemorrhage

This takes place by the self-sealing coagulation of blood in the opening of the cut vessels and in arteries this is aided by the contraction of the muscular walls of the severed vessel. In certain diseases, such as haemophilia or jaundice, the coagulation mechanism of the blood is impaired.

When a lot of blood is lost suddenly, the general blood pressure falls and the remaining blood coagulates more readily. The dangers of the reduction of blood volume are counteracted by a general vasoconstriction of the peripheral blood vessels of the body to maintain supplies to the vital heart–lung–brain circulation.

Permanent arrest of haemorrhage

This takes place when the blood clot or thrombus is replaced by organized fibrous tissue during the general healing of the injured part.

Treatment. The *local treatment* of bleeding depends upon the type of haemorrhage and the position and extent of the injury.

Arterial haemorrhage

The immediate first-aid treatment of this dangerous condition is to apply firm finger or thumb, *digital*, pressure to the bleeding point, preferably protecting the wound from infection by a sterile gauze swab. If this fails the main artery to the injured part must be compressed against an underlying bone if possible. (Arterial haemorrhage from the tongue may be controlled by pulling the tongue forward and compressing the lingual arteries against the mandible.) Subsequent deliberate surgical treatment may involve suturing the wound or even gripping the bleeding vessel with artery forceps and then tying off the open end with a ligature.

Venous haemorrhage

This is controlled by direct digital or other pressure to the bleeding point for about 5 minutes.

Capillary haemorrhage

This is not usually severe and stops spontaneously in most cases.

Haemorrhage immediately following dental extraction can usually be controlled by not allowing the patient to rinse the mouth with water and getting him to bite on a firm, sterile pack for a few minutes so that the socket is filled with undisturbed blood clot. Where the bleeding persists it may be controlled by suturing the wound or by the use of haemostatic (coagulation-producing) drugs or resorbable haemostatic packs that can be introduced into the socket. When a vasoconstricting local anaesthetic has been used to infiltrate a region before surgery, reactionary haemorrhage can occur when the effect wears off. Other common causes of post-extraction bleeding include excessive mouth washing, very hot food and drink, alcohol and excessive bodily activity during the recovery period.

First-aid treatment of post-extraction bleeding. The patient should be reassured, a cold mouth wash may be given to help remove excessive blood clots from other regions of the mouth, the bleeding point located and the patient given a sterile pack to bite on while the dental surgeon is called.

FAINTING (SYNCOPE)

This is the commonest general complication to occur in the dental surgery. However, the first signs and symptoms of this condition are similar to those of the more serious emergencies of respiratory failure, circulatory collapse and heart failure and the diagnosis of fainting may only be confirmed when the patient begins to respond to simple first-aid treatment.

Fainting may be caused by an unpleasant sensation such as severe pain, or emotional stimulation such as fear or surprise, and may be more likely to occur in a hot, airless atmosphere or as a result of severe haemorrhage. It is due to the overreaction of the vasomotor centres in the brain, which control the blood pressure, so that blood is diverted to the peripheral circulation and the brain is deprived of blood. The signs and symptoms are those of lack of oxygen to the brain. The patient feels distressed, weak, dizzy and nauseated. The skin becomes pale, sweaty and cold. The pulse rate is rapid and thin and the patient either shows signs of brain stimulation or depression. The pallor and sweating increase and the patient loses consciousness. The blood pressure falls and the pulse slows. The continued reduction of oxygen to the brain may cause involuntary muscle-twitching or even convulsions.

Treatment
1. At the first sign of fainting the patient should be placed in a horizontal position. If he is in a dental chair this may be tilted so that the head and heart are at a lower level than the legs. In this way the blood pressure to the brain is immediately raised by gravity.
2. Tight clothing around the neck should be loosened.
3. If consciousness is lost, administer oxygen by mask until the patient's colour returns to normal.
4. If recovery does not occur within a few minutes a more serious condition must be suspected and medical aid should be called. The patient's pulse and respiration rate should be kept under constant observation.

RESPIRATORY FAILURE
All respiration may stop and the patient will rapidly become *cyanosed* with blue lips and oral mucosa as the heart continues to circulate inadequately oxygenated blood through the body.

Treatment
1. Place the patient flat on his back on a firm surface, preferably the floor, checking his colour, chest movements and the carotid pulse.
2. Put the patient's head well back, drawing the jaw forward and supporting it. This brings the tongue forward, clear of the airway and may be all that is required to start the patient breathing again. Loosen any tight clothing at the patient's neck.
3. Clear the air passages of nose, mouth and throat. If the patient has loose dentures, remove them; if not, leave them in place as they help to give the mouth a better shape making artificial respiration easier.
4. **Mouth-to-mouth respiratory resuscitation** (Fig. 18/1). Inspire fully, place your mouth over the patient's mouth, sealing your lips around his mouth, pinch his nostrils closed with your fingers. Blow forcibly into his

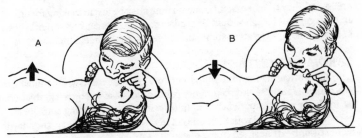

Fig. 18/1 Mouth-to-mouth resuscitation: A. inspiration; B. expiration

lungs, and watch the patient's chest expand each time – it should rise as the air enters the lungs.

5. **Mouth-to-nose respiratory resuscitation.** Inspire fully, place your mouth over the patient's nose, hold his jaw forward but close his mouth. Blow forcibly into the patient's lungs, and watch the patient's chest expand each time – it should rise as the air enters the lungs.

6. With either of these methods, mouth-to-mouth, or mouth-to-nose, raise your body and breathe in again while the patient expires passively.

7. Inspire deeply and repeat the sequence. Give the first two inflations as soon as possible then check the pulse to make sure that the heart is beating. If it is then continue to give inflations at a rate of 12 to 16 times a minute, continuing until the patient starts to breathe again, or help arrives.

If the chest does not expand after applying artificial respiration as described, it must be assumed that there is a blockage in the airway, and the oropharynx should be checked by sweeping it clear with a finger. If the blockage persists, other methods of dislodging it should be tried rapidly:

1. Roll the patient on his side (a child may be inverted over the forearm) and deliver several firm blows with the heel of the hand to the spine between the shoulder blades.

2. Use the *Heimlich manoeuvre* as follows: roll the patient onto his stomach (prone), straddle the lower torso, clasp both hands beneath the patient to form a fist in the mid-line and midway between the ribs and the naval and, in a sudden, rapid movement upward cause a rise in the pressure in the lungs that should expel any foreign body; resume artificial respiration.

Persistent blockage requires tracheostomy (where the surgeon makes an incision into the trachea to provide an accessory airway).
Note: Special airways, for example Brook airway, are made to conduct air from the operator to the patient without actual physical contact between the two. The Ambu-bag may also be used to inflate the lungs using only manual

pressure. They are not essential and no time must be lost in looking for one in an emergency. Oxygen should be available and the dental surgeon may wish to administer a respiratory stimulant to the patient by injection.

CARDIAC ARREST

The signs of cardiac failure and circulatory collapse may swiftly follow the loss of consciousness and respiratory failure. No pulse will be felt at the wrist or in the neck, the patient's condition will be deteriorating and he will become cold and grey with the pupils of his eyes dilated. No heart sound will be heard or heart beat felt in the chest.

Cardiac arrest need not be fatal if oxygenated blood can be pumped to the brain within 3 minutes, after which time permanent brain damage will occur.

Treatment

Note: External cardiac compression should not be carried out unless you are sure that the heart has stopped beating.

1. Note the time and call for help.
2. Place the patient flat on his back on a firm surface, preferably the floor.
3. Kneel alongside the patient facing his chest and in line with his heart.
4. Start external cardiac compression (Fig. 18/2). Find the junction of his

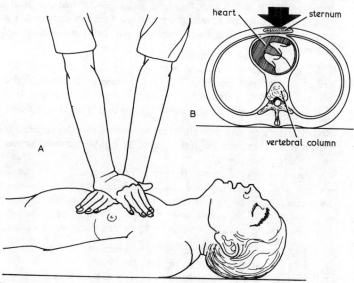

Fig. 18/2 A. Position of the hands on the sternum for external cardiac compression. B. Transverse section of the thorax

rib margins at the bottom of the breastbone (sternum). Place the heel of one hand along the line of the breastbone, about two finger-breadths above this point, keeping your fingers off the ribs. Cover this hand with the heel of your other hand and interlock your fingers. In children light pressure with one hand is sufficient.

5. With arms straight and your shoulders directly over the patient's breastbone, press down vertically about 4cm (1½in.), thus compressing the heart against the back wall of the chest.
6. Release the pressure and repeat (the sequence) at the rate of 60 to 80 compressions a minute.
7. An assistant should give mouth-to-mouth artificial respiration at the same time (see treatment of respiratory failure, p.218).
8. If the operator is alone give about 15 cardiac compressions, followed by two rapid lung inflations, and then repeat.
9. Continue the sequence until the patient is either out of danger, arrives at hospital or the patient's muscles stiffen from rigor mortis which indicates that death has occurred.

EMERGENCY KIT

This should contain the following drugs and agents, and the means to administer them quickly and efficiently. Such means will include: syringes and needles; ampoules of sterile water for injection (used to dissolve doses of dry drug powder also in sterile ampoules); skin cleaning swabs in tear-open sachets.

Airways, mouth-gags, tongue forceps, swabs, adequate suction apparatus, torch or pen-light.

Oxygen. This relieves anoxia due to shock, cardiac or respiratory failure. The high pressure from the cylinder must be lessened by a reducing valve and the gas administered with a mask.

Adrenaline (1:1000 solution). This is a circulatory and cardiac stimulant given by injection. It is also used in severe drug sensitivity reaction.

Hydrocortisone sodium succinate (for injection). This is used in the treatment of circulatory collapse or severe drug sensitivity reaction.

Antihistamines. These are used in the treatment of drug sensitivity reaction, such as penicillin sensitivity.

Glyceryl trinitrate (tablets). These are used for treating angina attacks.

Glucose. This is to treat hypoglycaemia.

A standard first aid box for treatment of simple cuts, scalds, burns, etc., plus a *first aid manual* are also essential.

CALLING AN AMBULANCE

Dial 999 from the nearest telephone and ask for the ambulance service. Give your telephone number first (in case you are cut off), then all details as clearly and quickly as possible. Only replace the receiver after the ambulance control officer does so – in case he needs more information.

CHAPTER NINETEEN

Care and Use of Drugs in Dentistry

A wide range of drugs is used in the local and general treatment of dental diseases. Some are kept immediately available for use in the dental surgery, while others, for the patient's home use, are supplied by the pharmacist in accordance with the dental surgeon's prescription or written order.

The DSA must always remember that all matters concerned with drugs need great responsibility on her part because of the powerful nature of many preparations and the dangers that can occur if they are carelessly handled or inappropriately administered.

MEDICINES LEGISLATION

The sale and supply of medicinal substances are controlled by the Medicines Act 1968. The Act divides these substances into three main classes:

1. *General sale list medicines* (GSL). These are medicinal products which can, with reasonable safety, be sold or supplied otherwise than under the supervision of a pharmacist.

2. *Pharmacy medicines* (P). These are any medicinal product which can only be sold or supplied from a pharmacy, for example, aspirin, paracetamol and codeine tablets. The Misuse of Drugs Act 1971 provides comprehensive control over drugs of all kinds and prohibits certain activities regarding manufacture, supply and possession of controlled drugs – those which are known to cause addiction or drug dependence if misused. The Misuse of Drugs Regulations 1973 defines the classes of person authorized to supply and possess controlled drugs while acting in their professional capacities and lays down conditions under which these activities may be carried out. Controlled drugs are listed in schedules which define the rigour of control of prescribing. For example, schedule 2 includes the main addictive drugs such as the opiates (heroin, morphine and methadone).

3. *Prescription only medicines* (POM). These are medicinal products including controlled drugs that may only be sold or supplied from pharmacies in accordance with a prescription given by a registered practitioner. (A pre-

scription is a written order from a doctor or dentist for the supply of drugs to a patient.)

A dental surgeon may keep in stock and administer certain controlled drugs, but only in so far as is necessary for the practice of his profession. If he does use such drugs in his practice he is required by law to keep a record of their receipt which should include:

1. The date on which the drug was received.
2. The name and address of the person or firm from whom it was received.
3. The amount received.
4. The form in which it was received.

These details should be recorded in a book set aside for this purpose. It is also advisable to record the occasions on which the controlled drug was administered, that is, the quantity and date. Controlled drugs must be stored in a locked, fixed receptacle for which the practitioner alone has the key. A dental surgeon is not authorized to supply these drugs other than by direct administration to a patient receiving dental treatment. However, he may prescribe such drugs for use outside the dental surgery for 'dental treatment only'.

The Dental Practitioners' Formulary (DPF) lists all the drugs and preparations that may be prescribed under the National Health Service in Britain. Since 1984 the DPF has been published in one volume together with the *British National Formulary* (BNF) which is the handbook for medical prescribing and allows the dental surgeon to identify drugs, and their actions, that patients may already be taking for general medical treatment. It is revised twice-yearly and is distributed free to all NHS practitioners.

Regulations for the control of drugs may be modified and amended from time to time and the latest details are to be found in *Medicines and Poisons Guide* published by The Pharmaceutical Press, 1 Lambeth High Street, London SE1 7JN.

CARE OF DRUGS IN THE DENTAL SURGERY

Records
As well as the controlled drugs records required by law, an accurate record of the dates and quantities of other drugs received at the practice should be maintained. This not only keeps track of the drugs, but will also be of help in reordering new stock by indicating the rate at which individual items are used up.

Storage and security
1. All drugs must be clearly labelled at all times and in case of doubt the unidentified drug should be destroyed.

2. All drugs should be stored in cool, dry conditions. Always check the manufacturer's advice about storage conditions and make a note on the label of the expiry date of preparations that are known to deteriorate on keeping.

3. Poisons must be clearly labelled by name, plus a cautionary label marked 'Poison' together with any warning notices, for example, 'This substance is caustic'. Poisonous liquids should be in ribbed bottles that are recognizable by touch. Poisons should be stored in a special cupboard, drawer or even a special shelf so that they are not mistaken for non-poisonous drugs. They must not be stored near foodstuffs.

4. Controlled drugs (see Misuse of Drugs Regulations, p.223) must be kept under the dental surgeon's personal supervision in a fixed, locked receptacle to which he alone has the key. This category of drugs is rarely required in general practice.

5. Analgesics, sedatives, hypnotics, tranquillizers and all drugs that act on the central nervous system are capable of producing a state of drug dependence or addiction in subjects to whom they are administered repeatedly and in sufficient dose. All such drugs should be kept under lock and key to avoid unauthorized use, as should the prescription pad. Theft of drugs is a matter of serious concern, and every precaution must be taken to prevent it.

6. Certain drugs, such as local anaesthetic solutions, penicillin, can cause hypersensitivity in members of the dental team if they are handled carelessly, even minute amounts, if they are allowed to come into frequent, unnecessary contact with the skin.

7. Caustic drugs, etc., for example, etchants, bleach solutions, can burn the skin if they are spilt. Containers should be handled with great care and must not be stored on high shelves where an accident could splash them into the face and eyes.

ADMINISTRATION OF DRUGS

The DSA must never give a drug to a patient, not even an aspirin, without the dental surgeon's direct instruction to do so on each occasion.

Drugs may be administered to the patient by various routes.

1. Oral. This is perhaps the commonest route. The drug is taken by mouth and absorbed from the gastrointestinal tract (for example, aspirin).

2. Sublingual. The drug is placed under the tongue and is absorbed through the oral mucosa (for example, glyceryl trinitrate in an angina pectoris attack). This route is rarely used in dentistry.

3. Intramuscularly, by injection into muscle (for example, penicillin).

4. Intravenously, by injection into a vein (for example, anaesthetic drugs).

5. Subcutaneously, by injection just beneath the skin (for example, local anaesthetic infiltration).
6. Inhalation, breathed in and absorbed by the lungs (for example, inhalation anaesthesia).
7. Topically, by application to the surface of the skin or tooth (for example, topical anaesthetic ointment).

WEIGHTS AND MEASURES

Doses of drugs are calculated and expressed by the metric system:
Weight

   1000 milligrams (mg) = 1 gram (g)
   1000 grams　　　　　= 1 kilogram (kg)

Volume

   1000 millilitres (ml) = 1 litre
   1 litre is the volume of 1 kilogram of water

The strength of a solution can be expressed as a percentage, for example:
1g weight or 1ml volume in 100ml water = a 1 per cent solution
5g weight or 5ml volume in 100ml water = a 5 per cent solution

SOME DRUGS USED IN DENTISTRY

Drugs are the substances or agents that are used in the treatment or prevention of disease and to assist the healing of wounds. They can be classified according to their action and uses.

Anaesthetics
See Chapter 12.

Analeptics
These drugs, for example, nikethamide, stimulate the respiratory centres and the central nervous system. They are usually given in the event of respiratory failure.

Analgesics
Mild analgesics (anodynes). These are drugs which relieve pain without causing loss of consciousness or sensation (feeling).

   Aspirin is used to relieve pain due to infection or injury, for headache and, because of its antipyretic (fever-reducing) action, it may be taken to alleviate the symptoms of a feverish cold. It may cause gastric irritation or bleeding if taken on an empty stomach and tablets should therefore be taken after meals, crushed or dissolved in water (soluble aspirin is available). Aspirin should not be given to children under the age of 12 years because of possible links with Reye's syndrome (a severe illness involving the brain, liver, etc.).

Paracetamol is also an analgesic antipyretic used to control mild or moderate pain, and it does not seem to cause indigestion or gastric bleeding. It is, however, more dangerous than aspirin in overdosage (as little as 20 tablets) because it can cause severe liver and kidney damage.

Dihydrocodeine (DF118) is a most potent and effective analgesic given by mouth. It may cause nausea and giddiness.

Codeine is a drug obtained from opium, but without its potent effects. It is usually taken in combination with aspirin or paracetamol in a tablet.

Strong analgesics. These include *morphine* (an opium derivative) and *pethidine*, drugs capable of relieving pain and producing a sense of well-being (euphoria) and mental detachment, which makes them potentially habit-forming drugs of dependence. They are not often used in general dental practice.

Antibiotics
These are drugs either synthetic or themselves derived from living organisms or moulds, which are capable of killing or inhibiting the growth of certain bacteria in the body. They are of great value in the treatment of severe infections in conjunction with standard surgical methods, for example, the drainage of abscesses. In certain conditions, for example, the presence of heart valve lesions after rheumatic fever, they may be given to prevent postoperative infective complications. Sensitization to certain antibiotics, especially penicillin, can occur both to patients under treatment and to anyone else handling the drug without proper care. Such sensitivity can cause skin rashes and bronchial spasm and even anaphylactic shock upon further exposure to the drug and these unpleasant and even dangerous effects have to be treated with antihistamine drugs or adrenaline injections.

Penicillin is the most effective antibiotic. It may be administered by injection intramuscularly or by buffered oral preparations. No patient must be given penicillin without first asking them if they have any previous history of sensitivity to the drug. Ampicillin and amoxycillin are semi-synthetic penicillins.

Tetracycline is a broad-spectrum antibiotic effective against a wide range of bacteria, usually given orally for general infections. Tetracycline mouth baths are used for primary herpetic stomatitis. If this drug is taken during the period of tooth mineralization it may be deposited in the calcifying areas and cause discoloration.

Erythromycin is sometimes used to treat infections in patients who are sensitive to penicillin (see fungicides, p.231).

Metronidazole (Flagyl) is an antibacterial drug which has a high activity against certain anaerobic bacteria. It is used effectively in oral Vincent's infection (AUG).

Anticoagulants

These are taken in certain medical conditions, such as heart disease, to prevent blood clotting in the blood vessels, for example, heparin, warfarin, etc.

Antidepressants

These are drugs, for example, *monoamine-oxidase inhibitors (MAOI)* and *lithium* given to relieve depressive illness. Patients taking MAOI drugs may suffer a dangerous rise in blood pressure if they eat certain foods (cheese, marmite, broad beans, etc.), or if they are given a drug which interacts with the antidepressant, for example, pethidine, morphine or a local anaesthetic containing noradrenaline.

Antihistamines

These are drugs used in the treatment of skin rashes and other reactions caused by sensitivity to certain substances, such as penicillin. They include *chlorpheniramine maleate* (Piriton) and *promethazine hydrochloride* (Phenergan). These drugs themselves may have side-effects causing dry mouth and drowsiness.

Antiseptics and disinfectants

Antiseptics are substances which inhibit or arrest the growth and multiplication of bacteria. *Disinfectants* destroy bacteria but cannot be relied upon to kill spores and viruses (see Chapter 5). '*Germicides*' kill 'germs'. Most antiseptics may be applied to living tissues without causing injury, but disinfectant is the term usually applied to agents destroying pathogenic organisms and used for large-scale disinfection of inanimate objects.

Instruments and utensils may be disinfected by boiling them in water (100°C) for 15 minutes.

Alcohol. A 60 to 95 per cent solution is rapidly bactericidal and a 70 per cent solution is an antiseptic used for cleaning intact skin before injections or working surfaces in the surgery (surgical spirit, industrial methylated spirit).

Aldehydes. Formaldehyde (as formalin solution) is a strong disinfectant that is irritant to the skin. A 2 per cent solution is germicidal after 30 minutes and a 4 to 8 per cent solution may kill spores after 24 hours. Formaldehyde vapour has a very slow sterilizing action.

Glutaraldehyde is an alkaline solution which is claimed to be a rapid sporicide (that is, it kills organisms and their spores) and is suitable for surface sterilization. Hard-surfaced, non-absorbent instruments should be totally immersed in a 2 per cent activated solution for 3 hours (8 to 10 hours is safer). All the solution must be washed off with sterile water.

Paraformaldehyde, a solid polymer which slowly releases formalin at body temperature, is a tissue-fixing agent used in pulp mummification. This toxic material has to be used with care to prevent it from escaping from the tooth.

Formolsaline solution is used to store biopsy material before it is examined in the laboratory.

Dyes. Solutions of certain dyes act as mild antibacterial agents, for example, crystal violet, brilliant green. They are rarely used in dentistry.

Halogens. A dilute solution of *iodine* may sometimes be used as an antiseptic and its stain indicates the area of application.

Iodoform, occurs as yellow crystals, which slowly liberate iodine. It is used as an antiseptic agent to treat infected wounds and in certain root canal therapy agents. BIPP (bismuth, iodoform and paraffin paste) is an ointment used on ribbon gauze to dress extraction sockets.

Chlorine. 1 per cent sodium hypochlorite solution (Milton) is a non-toxic antiseptic and germicide. It may be used to irrigate root canals. A 2 per cent solution is used to disinfect surfaces and equipment. Stronger solutions of the hypochlorite are caustic and also act as bleaching solutions.

Chlorhexidine (Hibitane) is a halogen compound used for skin cleansing and in hand cleansers (Hibiscrub). It is also used in aqueous solutions and gels to inhibit plaque formation.

Oxidizing agents. *Hydrogen peroxide* has antiseptic, deodorant and bleaching properties. It is regarded as a weak germicide of short duration. A 20 volume solution, diluted 1:20 with water, is used as a mouthwash and as a debris-removing agent in root canal therapy ('20 volume' means that 20 volumes of oxygen can be released from 1 volume of the solution).

Phenols and cresols (and their derivatives). *Phenol* (carbolic acid) is a strong disinfectant and protoplasmic poison. Pure phenol and strong solutions are caustic and can rapidly penetrate and kill skin and mucous membranes. If absorbed further into the body it is extremely toxic and affects the central nervous system. The local antidote is to wash the affected body surface with alcohol and then apply glycerin to the burn.

A 1 per cent phenol solution is a disinfectant but is rarely used on the tissues because of the danger of absorption into the body.

A 5 per cent phenol solution is a disinfectant but cannot be relied upon to kill spores.

Carbolized resin is used to devitalize the dental pulp.

Monochlorophenol with *camphor* is used as a root canal disinfectant.

Cresol (tricresol) is a disinfectant used in root canal therapy.

Thymol is a phenolic disinfectant used in mouthwashes.

Hexachloraphane: soaps and creams containing 1 to 3 per cent are used to reduce the bacterial flora on the skin. It should not be applied repeatedly to the whole surface of the body (*particularly in infants*).

Creosote is derived from tar. It acts as a mild local analgesic and antiseptic and is used in pulp therapy and root canal treatment.

Eugenol is the essential constituent of clove oil (clove oil contains 85 to 90 per cent of eugenol). It has an antiseptic and obtundent action and is used with zinc oxide powder as a basis of many temporary filling materials and gingival packs. It may be used as an antiseptic in pulp and root canal therapy.

Surface active agents. Benzalkonium chloride (Roccal, Zephiran (USA)) is a quaternary ammonium compound and forms non-irritant, detergent, antiseptic and disinfectant solutions. A 0.1 per cent solution can be used for preoperative cleaning and disinfection of the skin.

Cetrimide (Cetavlon): a 0.5 per cent in 70 per cent alcohol solution is used for preoperative disinfection of the skin. An aqueous solution of 1 per cent can be used for cleaning utensils.

Chlorhexidine agents. Chlorhexidine (Hibitane) as a 1 per cent solution can be used for preoperative disinfection of the skin. Dilute solutions can be used as a mouthwash.

Antitoxins

These are substances which counteract bacterial toxins (for example, tetanus toxoid).

Antiviral agents

New synthetic agents are being developed to combat viral diseases.

Idoxuridine (0.1 per cent) is used locally to treat herpes ulceration in the eye, but is seldom needed for oral infection because of its toxicity.

Acyclovir (Zovirax) may be used locally and systemically to treat herpes simplex.

Caustics

These are substances that cause local burns or tissue death (for example, phenol).

Corticosteroids

These are products of the adrenal cortex (a ductless gland). Their action is to modify tissue reactions to injury and inflammation by suppressing the disease function and they have an effect on the general circulation and blood pressure. They are used topically in the form of *hydrocortisone sodium succinate* lozenges (Corlan Pellets) and creams, *triamcinolone acetonide* paste (Adcortyl-A in Orabase), in the treatment of aphthous ulceration of the mouth.

Patients under medical treatment with steroids for general diseases such as arthritis and chronic skin diseases are likely to suffer severe shock and collapse during routine anaesthesia and surgery unless they are protected by an increased preoperative dose of the drug given in direct consultation with their medical adviser. *Hydrocortisone sodium succinate* injection is used to treat the sudden onset of anaphylactic shock and circulatory collapse (see Chapter 18).

Emetics
These include drugs such as ipecacuanha given to induce vomiting (emesis) in order to empty the stomach as part of the emergency treatment of certain types of poisoning.

Fungicides
These kill fungi and moulds; *fungistats* inhibit their growth. They are used in the treatment of thrush, 'denture sore mouth', and occasionally in root canal therapy.

Nystatin is used topically in the form of tablets which are allowed to dissolve in the mouth.

Amphotericin B (Fungilin) is used in the same way but has a less unpleasant taste.

Haemostatics
These are drugs and measures that arrest bleeding.

Physical measures. These are pressure, pack, suture.

Absorbable haemostatics. Oxidized cellulose gauze (*surgicel*) is used dry in the wound and, with the escaping blood, forms an artificial clot. Fibrin foam and bone wax are also used.

Vasoconstrictors. The adrenaline in local anaesthetic solution causes constriction of the capillaries and reduces local bleeding.

Hypnotics, sedatives and tranquillizers
Narcotics. These are drugs which depress the central nervous system (hypnotics and sedatives, for example). Great care should be exercised in the provision of these drugs to ensure that the patient does not become

dependent upon them. In dentistry they may be considered to be a rare, 'one-off' requirement.

Hypnotics. These are drugs which induce sleep.

Nitrazepam may be given the night before a dental operation to ensure a good night's sleep. The after-effects include delayed reaction times the next day.

Chloral hydrate is often used for children and lasts about 8 hours. Triclofos is similar to chloral hydrate but is less irritant to the stomach and can be given in tablet or syrup form.

Sedatives. These depress the central nervous system, have a mood-calming effect and soothe the anxious patient. They also dull the faculties and make the patient sleepy so that he is unable to carry out his normal activity. They reduce preoperative apprehension if given an hour or so beforehand.

Diazepam (Valium) and *chloral hydrate* act as sedatives in subhypnotic doses.

Tranquillizers. These give the patient 'peace of mind'. They have a calming effect without impairing the patient's alertness. They are often taken for long periods, under careful medical supervision. Their effectiveness varies widely in different patients. *Chlordiazepoxide* (Librium) and *diazepam* (Valium) are probably the best-known tranquillizers.

Note: Patients taking these drugs must not attempt to drive a car or work machinery. They must not take alcohol, which potentiates the action of the drug.

Medical gas cylinders
The following are labelling and identification colours for medical gas cylinders, British Standard, 1955.

Gas		Shoulder	Body
Oxygen	O_2	White	Black
Nitrous oxide	N_2O	Blue	Blue
Oxygen and carbon dioxide mixture	O_2+CO_2	White and grey	Black
Air		White and black	Grey

The name of the gas is stencilled on the body of each cylinder and is also clearly stamped on the metal cylinder valve.

Oxygen is stored at high pressure (140 bar, 2000lb/in²) and has to be regulated with a reducing valve. This gas, although not inflammable itself, makes things burn more readily. Take care to avoid smoking or electric sparks from apparatus, etc., where pure oxygen is being used.

Mummifying agents
These kill tissues and render them resistant to subsequent growth of organisms. They are used in certain forms of pulp therapy, especially in deciduous teeth. They include *formaldehyde, paraformaldehyde, iodoform* and *cresol*.

Obtundents
These are drugs used locally to dull the sensitivity of dentine during excavation of a cavity. They include *eugenol, phenol* and *cresol*.

Emergency kit
See Chapter 18, p.221.

CHAPTER TWENTY

Study Methods and Examination Technique

It is always easier to settle down to the continuous attainment of knowledge over a prolonged period if this is being done to achieve some specific end. From the outset a constantly growing and expanding knowledge of dentistry will make your everyday work far more interesting and worthwhile, but if you are also preparing to take a recognized professional examination for dental surgery assistants you know that every moment of study is taking you nearer to a most important personal achievement. To have gained a qualification of this sort brings considerable satisfaction and self-confidence and will give you status in personal advancement and future job applications.

Anyone who has the normal curiosity and interest about their work is capable of getting down to study and, if you go about it in an organized and planned way, there is a great deal of enjoyment to be gained from the sense of purpose that is quickly felt. Planned study can be carried out with an increasing economy of effort as your mind becomes accustomed to the habits of observing, remembering and thinking to some definite purpose.

Before setting out on a course of study you are recommended to discuss the matter with your own dental surgeon. You can also obtain valuable advice by writing to your national examining board for details of their examination, their syllabus of study and copies of recent examination papers. You should also contact local colleges or dental schools for particulars of their DSA courses.

THEORETICAL AND PRACTICAL TUITION

Several methods of tuition are available:

1. Full-time courses at dental schools or day colleges.
2. Part-time evening or other classes at colleges.
3. Private coaching.
4. Correspondence courses.
5. Self-tuition.

As well as theoretical knowledge the trained DSA must also have a considerable amount of practical chairside experience that can only be gained in the dental surgery assisting the dental surgeon – who is thus the most important teacher you will have.

Most people find it stimulating to attend a regular course of lectures and classes. There is help, encouragement and enthusiasm from the teacher and a chance to measure your own standards against those of the other students. However, your teacher cannot learn the facts for you and the main effort of study still lies in organized, planned self-tuition, day by day.

STUDY METHODS

From the start allocate a certain amount of time each day for study and make sure that you keep to it rigidly. It is important not to be too ambitious about this time allocation. One hour a day at first will be ample. Small amounts of work, regularly carried out, will achieve a great effect. Try to choose a time of day when you will be feeling fresh and alert. You will soon get into the study habit.

Make out two timetables, one the long-term strategical plan of work which will divide up the total course, and the other a short-term tactical timetable for the next week or so. The latter means that you will soon feel the stimulating satisfaction, gained by achieving working targets and deadlines, that is so important in maintaining a long-term planned effort. In the long-term timetable make sure that you leave some margins of time for unpredictable events such as holidays, illness and so on. Make sure that you have some completely free time in your timetable for rest and recreation. When you reach the point of being able to study for more than an hour at a time, take 5 minutes' rest away from your work every hour; even this short break will refresh your mind considerably.

Try to find the best place and conditions for your study periods. The things that you *must* have are a desk or a table, a comfortable chair (but not too comfortable!), adequate light, heating and ventilation in a room that is reasonably quiet. Keep your books and study things together so that you can start each period of study without having the delay or distraction of time-wasting preparation. Tell your family and friends that you are studying and the hours that you have set aside for it. This will strengthen your resolve to get down to work (you won't want to let yourself down!) and also stop them from unwittingly interrupting your new work habits.

Remember that there are many odd moments during the day that can also be used for study and revision. For example, the time spent in public transport on the journey to and from work and spare minutes during the lunch break can be used to your advantage if you always carry a book, journal or notes about with you.

Notebooks

It is important to keep clear and accurate written notes of your studies, limiting them to essential facts and principles. This will give the immediate benefit of a sense of progress and achievement; it will practice the important arts of understanding and organizing facts and writing them down; it will improve your spelling and handwriting and, most valuable of all, you will be assembling your notes for pre-examination revision. These notes are best kept in a looseleaf file.

A second pocket notebook can be carried at all times so that you can make an immediate note of items that you come across during the working day that are worthy of adding to your best looseleaf file later on. Lecture notes may also be taken down quickly in a rough book and then copied out carefully into the file as soon as possible for this is a very effective method of early revision. Watch out for the correct spelling of unfamiliar words heard in lectures.

Reading

Reading forms an important part of your studies and you should develop a new technique if you are to get the most help possible from a book. First of all do not be daunted by the length of it or try to get through a certain number of pages each day. Start by skimming through the whole book trying to see the shape of it all, how the chapters are laid out and the broad outline of what its author is trying to convey to you. Then go back to the beginning and read it in detail at the rate you find most suitable, making notes or underlining key words and sentences. Parts of it will seem more difficult and will need more time, others will go quickly. Finally, read the whole thing through again in the light of your own growing personal knowledge and experience. All the time try to carry any new facts into the dental surgery with you to test and perhaps relate them to your everyday practical work. Get your dental surgeon to discuss them with you – most dentists love to talk about their work to an intelligent and enquiring audience!

Borrow dental journals and keep an eye on current trends and materials. In free moments talk to the dental technician, the oral hygienist, the anaesthetist, the other dental surgery assistants and the dental company representatives about dentistry for they are all valuable sources of information. Very few people will resent such curiosity and most will be flattered that you have asked them.

Revision

General revision should be carried out currently during the whole period of study and not left entirely until the last week or two before the examination. Make sure that your timetable allows you to go back and read through your notes at frequent intervals. Diligent, methodical work will mean that little intensive revision is required and will play its part in reducing pre-examination tensions. You should test yourself frequently from the outset of your studies to make sure that you can remember important lists of facts. This is best done by actively reciting them from memory or writing them down, rather than passively reading them through. Make up mnemonics to help you to recall long lists of facts by constructing a sentence or word using the initial letters of the facts in question (for example, the branches of the external carotid artery: *S*uperior thyroid, *L*ingual, *F*acial, *O*ccipital, ascending *P*haryngeal, posterior *A*uricular, *S*uperficial temporal and *M*axillary can be recalled from the mnemonic '*S*ome *L*ittle *F*ellows *O*pen *P*urses *A*nd *S*teal *M*oney').

Self-testing can be extended by working through questions from old examination papers. This will help you to gain further practice in expressing yourself in writing and will train you up to the standard of being able to write for a prolonged period in the actual examination.

Pre-examination

Try to spend a restful day before the actual examination, though some people feel happier just glancing through their notebooks again. Get together all the things that you will need in the examination and work out the route to the examination hall. Go to bed early and try to put the affairs of the next day out of your mind.

EXAMINATION

On the morning of the examination get up early and have a good breakfast.

You will have collected together your 'Examination Kit':
A clean uniform and cap (plain shoes, no jewellery, neat hair style, clean fingernails, no nail varnish, discreet make-up and perfume) which will be worn for the practical and oral examination. Facilities for changing will be available at the examination centre.
Admission card
Fountain pen and refill, or ball-point pens
Pencils and sharpener   Coloured pencils
Rubber   Ruler   Watch

Arrive at the examination hall early. This will allow you to get settled and used to the surroundings. Remember that nervousness before an examination is universal. Some of the candidates like to 'unload' their tensions onto others, so be careful who you chum up with in the moments before the examination room doors are opened to you. Your own slight tension is good for you, although you may find it hard to believe. The stressed feeling can be used to give you that special elation that means that you will be able to do your best. Make that energy work for you by keeping cool and collected.

Nervousness on its own will not fail an examination, but bland over-confidence can do so.

Once in the examination room, settle down and take your time to read the paper through, taking particular care to read the examiner's instructions at the top of the page. Is the timing and the number of questions to be answered the same as in the previous papers you have practised on? Plan out how long you have to answer each question. Choose which essay questions you are going to answer and read them through again checking for the key words that precisely define the extent of the answer required. Jot down an outline of your answers – just main paragraph headings and fact lists. As you do this you will find that your previously despised tension will have your mind working faster than you thought possible and ideas and facts will come rushing from your memory just as you need them.

Now you can start to write out your answers. Start off with the easiest question first, keep your answer simple and with the examiner in mind as if you were explaining it all to him. Get the points in order and make headings. Put in some simple drawings if they are appropriate and label them carefully. Try to set the whole thing out in a neat, attractive and legible style. It may be 'window-dressing' but examiners are human beings! Watch the time constantly for you must answer *all* the questions if you are to get good marks. If time presses before you can complete the answer to the last question at least jot down the headings for they can gain precious marks for you. The examiner is not trying to fail you so give him all the help you possibly can! Finally, read through your answers carefully. You'll be surprised at the number of punctuation and spelling mistakes you will have made.

In some cases part of the written examination is in the form of *multiple choice questions*. A printed questionnaire is provided which has spaces for the candidate to say which of the two or three alternative answers provided is correct or else to write in one-word or two-word answers. This is a pure test of knowledge and overcomes the difficulty that some people have in expressing themselves in essay questions. Work your way through the questions and if any of them hold you up leave them, complete all the easy questions first and then go back to the one or two that you find difficult. In this way you will not miss any opportunity to gain marks. There may also be short answer questions a diagram to be labelled and a charting test, as well as the essay type question in the second part of the written paper.

Between the paper and the practical and oral examination, if they are all on the same day, try to have a light, quiet meal and, if possible, a short walk in the fresh air.

In the oral and practical parts of the examination you will be given 'spotter' tests, practical tests and an oral examination. The 'spotter' test will ask you to identify and list by name and usage groups of dental instruments and materials. In the practical test you will be asked to carry out a specific technique, such as mixing an impression material and loading a tray, or mounting radiographs on a hanger. In the oral examination the examiner will spend a short time asking questions about all aspects of dentistry, both practical and theoretical.

In all this you must be aware constantly of the impression you are trying to make. This will be reflected in your dress, your posture, your manner and your voice. Remember to speak up always and even smile occasionally.

For further details, the intending student should consult the syllabus and regulations for the appropriate National Certificate of the Examining Board for Dental Surgery Assistants. This will include up-to-date details of the requirements for eligibility for entrance to the examination and information of what the examination includes. Copies of past examination papers are also available. In Britain such details for this national examination may be obtained from: The Association of Dental Surgery Assistants, DSA House, 29 London Street, Fleetwood, Lancashire FY7 6JY.

When you have passed the examination, do not be tempted to allow your study habit and knowledge to be neglected. Dentistry is constantly expanding. The trained dental surgery assistant owes it to herself and her profession to keep alert and up-to-date.

CHAPTER TWENTY-ONE

Examination Questions

The following represent a selection of the questions set in recent examination papers by the Examining Board for Dental Surgery Assistants for the National Certificate. They are reproduced by permission of the Board.

1. Describe briefly the main constituents of blood and their functions.
   What is the DSA's role in the treatment of post-extraction haemorrhage in the absence of the dentist?

2. List the different types of syringe that may be found in a dental surgery. Describe the uses of each.

3. What do you understand by the term 'viral hepatitis' and what are the problems associated with it?
   Discuss the management in the surgery of a known carrier.

4. A patient attends surgery for intravenous sedation.
   What are the duties of the DSA?

5. Write short notes on each of the following:
   a. Fissure sealants.
   b. The care of a removable orthodontic appliance.
   c. Dentine.

6. How should patients and staff be protected when dental radiographs are being taken?
   How would you process a film using a manual method?

7. Describe the methods used to prevent the occurrence of dental caries?

8. a. Why may teeth be splinted and what methods are used?
   What advice might you give to a patient who has been fitted with a splint?
   b. What is meant by pulpotomy?
   Say why this procedure is carried out.

9. Describe the duties of the DSA in maintaining a high standard of general cleanliness in the surgery and other patient areas.
   Suggest appropriate cleaning and disinfecting materials and their uses.

10. Describe the classification of malocclusion. Outline the methods by which malocclusion is treated. What advice would the DSA give to a patient wearing a fixed appliance?

11. Write short notes on the following:
   a. The care and maintenance of hand instruments following their use.

b. The inferior alveolar nerve (inferior dental nerve).

c. The disposal of hazardous waste materials.

12. Describe the non-clinical role of the dental surgery assistant in organizing and running an efficient practice system.

13. Describe the positions of the main salivary glands. What are the functions of saliva?

14. Why is moisture control important in dental procedures? What methods are available and what is the role of the DSA?

15. State the stages of construction of full upper and lower dentures. Describe your duties before, during and after each stage.

16. A patient is to have teeth extracted under general anaesthesia. List the instructions to be given to the patient, with reasons for each instruction:

a. When the appointment is made.

b. On the treatment visit.

What is the role of the DSA during the operation?

17. a. What are the signs and symptoms of acute inflammation?

b. Describe the process of dental caries leading to an acute abscess.

18. a. Name three handpieces and indicate the important features and uses of each.

b. How would you maintain them in good condition?

c. List the cutting instruments which may be used with them.

19. Describe with the aid of a diagram, the blood and nerve supply to the lower teeth. List the contents of a commonly used tube of local anaesthetic solution, giving the function of each constituent.

20. What would you do in the following situations?

a. A patient arrives stating that he has toothache following a recent filling done by another dentist.

b. A new patient age 15 attends for an extraction.

c. A patient arrives to have new dentures fitted, but says he has no money to pay.

d. An unaccompanied patient arrives by car for an extraction under general anaesthetic.

21. What procedures are carried out when:

a. A needle is fractured during a local anaesthetic injection?

b. A patient complains of feeling faint?

c. Bleeding is continuous after extraction?

d. The patient vomits whilst an impression is being taken?

22. a. Describe in detail a method with which you are familiar for the preparation of amalgam. What specific precautions would you take and why would you do so?

b. Briefly mention any other methods you know that are suitable for preparing amalgam.

242 *Examination Questions*

23. What is meant by an apicectomy? Why is it performed?
    How would the DSA assist during an apicectomy and retrograde root filling?
24. Write short notes on:
    a. The DSA's role in storage and handling of drugs.
    b. Immediate dentures.
25. Describe the preparation and uses of:
    a. Rubber base materials.
    b. Alginate.
    What precautions should be taken until the models are cast?

'SPOTTER' TESTS

Figs 21/1, 21/2, 21/3 and 21/4 show examples of instrument layouts for various procedures. The instruments are not named, but you can use these pictures to test your knowledge.

In each spotter the candidate is asked to identify in full 20 items, arranged in groups of four; 1 minute is allowed for each group. The candidate may pick up any item to examine it but must replace it carefully in its original position.

Specimen items

1. a. Double-ended excavator
   b. Gutta percha point
   c. Rubber mouth prop
   d. Flat-bladed plastic

2. a. Lower permanent molar forceps
   b. Sandpaper disc
   c. Amalgam plugger
   d. Impression syringe

3. a. Rongeurs
   b. Coupland's chisel
   c. Rubber Dam/clamp
   d. Gingival periodontal probe string

4. a. Ward's carver
   b. Occlusal x-ray film
   c. Bite-wing x-ray film
   d. Greenstick impression compound

5. a. Straight enamel chisel
   b. Cartridge syringe
   c. Articulating paper
   d. Composite mixing spatula

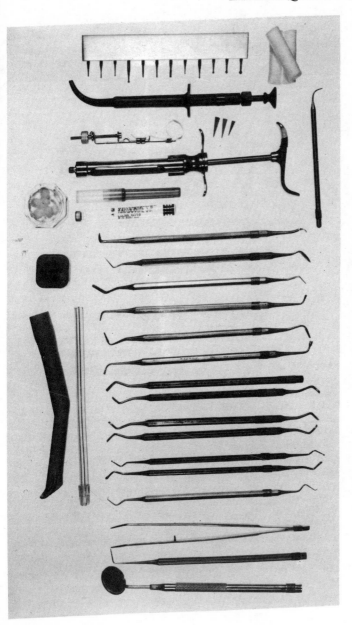

Fig. 21/1 Basic conservation tray

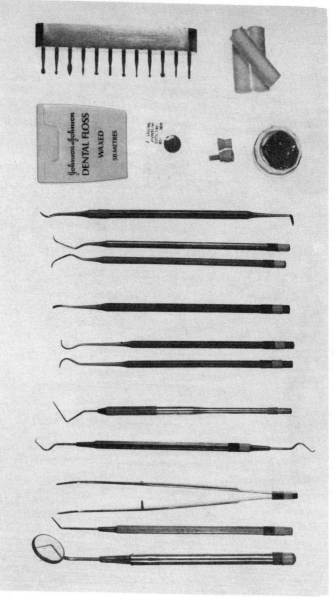

Fig. 21/2 Basic scale and polish tray

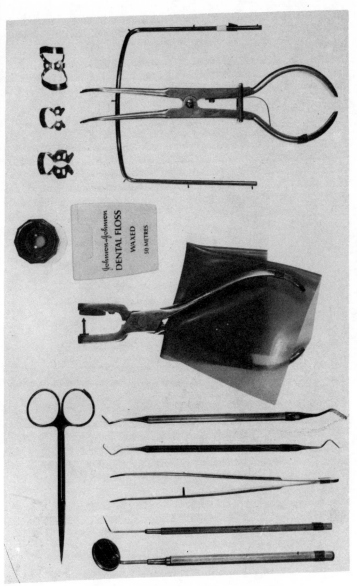

Fig. 21/3 Rubber Dam application tray

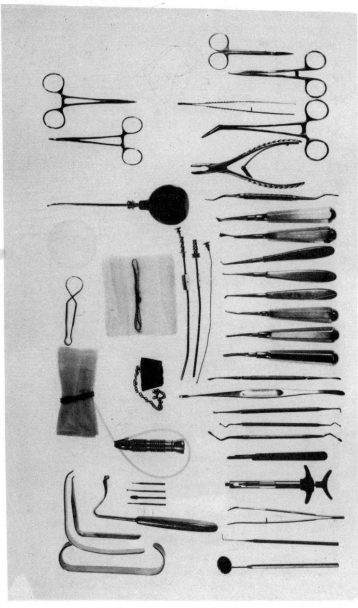

Fig. 21/4 Basic oral surgery trolley set up

Further Reading

Combe, E. C. (1986). *Notes on Dental Materials*, 5th edition. Churchill Livingstone, Edinburgh.

Dental Practitioner's Formulary (1986–88). British Dental Association, British Medical Association and the Pharmaceutical Society of Great Britain, London.

Erridge, P. L. (1988). *Self-Assessment Questions and Answers for Dental Assistants*, 2nd edition. John Wright, Bristol.

First Aid Manual (1987), 5th edition. St. John Ambulance, St. Andrew's Ambulance Association. The British Red Cross.

Forrest, J. O. (1981). *Preventive Dentistry*, 2nd edition. John Wright, Bristol.

Frommer, H. H. (1987). *Radiology for Dental Auxiliaries*, 4th edition. C. V. Mosby Co., St Louis.

Gelbier, S. and Copley, M. A. H. (1977). *Handbook for Dental Surgery Assistants and Other Ancillary Workers*, 2nd edition. John Wright, Bristol.

Gray's Anatomy, 36th edition (1981). Longman Group Limited, Edinburgh. (The sections relating to the teeth and jaws.)

Guide to Blood Borne Viruses and the Control of Cross Infection in Dentistry. Pamphlet published by the British Dental Association, London.

Harty, F. J. and Ogston, R. (1987). *Concise Illustrated Dental Dictionary*. John Wright, Bristol.

Kidd, E. A. M. and Joyston-Bechal (1987). *Essentials of Dental Caries: The Disease and its Management*. John Wright, Bristol.

Levison, H. (1982). *Textbook for Dental Nurses*, 5th edition. Blackwell Scientific Publications Limited, Oxford.

Maddox, Harry. *How to Study*. Pan Books, London.

Moore, J. R. and Gillbe, G. V. (1981). *Principals of Oral Surgery*, 3rd edition. Manchester University Press, Manchester.

Notes for Students of Dental Health Education. Health Education Authority Dental Health Publications Source List.

Pearce, E. (1975). *Anatomy and Physiology for Nurses*, 16th edition. Faber and Faber, London.

Smith, N. J. D. (1980). *Dental Radiography*. Blackwell Scientific Publications Limited, Oxford.
*Radiological Protection in Dental Practice**
*Emergencies in Dental Practice**

---

* These two pamphlets are published by the Department of Health, Richmond House, 79 Whitehall, London SW1A 2NS.

Index